Clinical Risk Modification: A Route to Clinical Governance?

Edited by

Jo Wilson MSc(Dist) PGDip BSc(Hons) MIPD
MHSM AIRM RGN RM RSCN

John Tingle BA Law(Hons) Cert Ed MEd Barrister

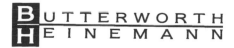

OXFORD   AUCKLAND   BOSTON   JOHANNESBURG   MELBOURNE   NEW DELHI

Butterworth-Heinemann
Linacre House, Jordan Hill, Oxford OX2 8DP
225 Wildwood Avenue, Woburn, MA 01801-2041
A division of Reed Educational and Professional Publishing Ltd

A member of the Reed Elsevier plc group

First published 1999

© Reed Educational and Professional Publishing Ltd 1999

British Library Cataloguing in Publication Data
A catalogue record for this book is available from the British Library

ISBN 0 7506 2939 8

1003110932

Typeset by BC Typesetting, Bristol
Printed and bound in Great Britain by Biddles Ltd, Guildford and King's Lynn

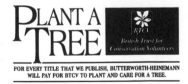

FOR EVERY TITLE THAT WE PUBLISH, BUTTERWORTH-HEINEMANN
WILL PAY FOR BTCV TO PLANT AND CARE FOR A TREE.

Contents

List of contributors

Paul Balen MA
Partner, Freeth Cartwright Hunt Dickins Solicitors, Nottingham, Leicester and Derby, UK

Pippa Bark BSc
Senior Research Fellow, Clinical Risk Unit, Psychology Department, University College London, UK

Cheryl Blundell LLB
Associate, Health Group, Bond Pearce Solicitors, Southampton, Bristol, Exeter, Plymouth, UK

Adrian Conduit FIMLS DipHSM MHSM MBA
Operations' Director, Clinical Services/Facilities, Birmingham Heartlands Hospital, UK

Lucy Frith BA, MPhil
Lecturer in Health Care Ethics, Department of Primary Care, University of Liverpool, Liverpool, UK

Bernadette Maughan BA
Nottingham Health Authority, Nottingham, UK

Thoreya Swage MBBS MA (Oxon)
Independent Consultant in Healthcare Management, Farnham, Surrey, UK

Dennis J. Van Liew MSc BSc
Director, Information, Healthcare Risk Resources International, London, UK

John Tingle BA Law(Hons) Cert Ed MEd Barrister
Reader in Health Law, The Nottingham Law School, Nottingham Trent University, Nottingham, UK

Jo Wilson MSc(Dist) PGDip BSc(Hons) MIPD MHSM AIRM RGN RM RSCN
Director, Clinical Consultancy, Healthcare Risk Resources International, Newcastle upon Tyne, UK

1 INTRODUCTION TO CLINICAL RISK MANAGEMENT AND MODIFICATION

Jo Wilson and John Tingle

INTRODUCTION

Healthcare costs have escalated so dramatically in the past few decades that the healthcare delivery system is presently under detailed scrutiny and is continually the target of reforms. These reforms bring with them organisational, clinical, business and financial risks which need to be identified, assessed and controlled to reduce unnecessary liability. Reforms require cultural and behaviour changes which take time to evolve and, if not properly managed, can increase uncertainty and risk exposure. Clinical risk modification addresses these exposures through a process of evolutionary development to minimise risk and maximise effective healthcare.

THE NHS REFORMS 1997

The Labour Government White Paper, *The New NHS, Modern, Dependable*, is the latest episode of change[1]. It brings a move away from the internal market and GP (general practitioner) fundholding and puts a renewed emphasis on promoting consistently high-quality clinical care and clinical effectiveness. Under the internal market, healthcare providers' primary statutory responsibility was financial in terms of balancing the books. System inefficiencies, process deficiencies, wasted resources, new technologies, consumer expectations, clinical negligence, iatrogenic injuries, litigation expenses, and a host of other factors have contributed to costs spiralling out of control. With the sweeping NHS reforms and the moves to a primary-care led NHS with primary care groups (PCGs) and primary care trusts, it is imperative that healthcare practitioners begin to demonstrate cost- and clinical effectiveness, evidence-based practice, and high-quality patient care.

PRIMARY-CARE LED NHS

The 1990s have been a time of moving the organisation of care towards a primary-care driven and led NHS. The 1989 White Paper, *Working for*

Patients, directly promoted GP fundholding, and indirectly encouraged locality commissioning and GP commissioning[2]. This led some groups of GPs to rally ahead and experiment with GP multifunds, fundholding consortia and total purchasing projects which are providing a much wider range of patient services and speedier access to secondary care. The role of many GPs changed from service provider to that of a purchaser and provider of services. Some GPs have welcomed and developed these changes while others have remained as non-fundholders under the control of their health authority, creating what is perceived as a two-tier system. Throughout all these changes GPs have retained their independent contractor status, having a contract with their health authority to provide general medical services to their local population. The 1996 White Paper, *Choice and Opportunity*, aimed to create more flexibility in providing and developing primary care services[3]. 1997 and 1998 brought the developments of locality commissioning pilot projects and schemes with the aim being to develop more locally sensitive services. The White Paper of 1997, *The New NHS, Modern, Dependable*, is a firm endorsement of the strengths and potential of developments in primary care and the establishment of primary care groups (PCGs)[1]. There are organisational and clinical risks inherent in these endorsements with too many questions being left unanswered and fears from secondary care specialists feeling that they will not have sufficient say and will become increasingly beholden to GPs. Others see it as a positive step in having clinical professionals, not health authorities, directly involved in commissioning services, moving away from the current two-tier system. The agenda has to be based on working in partnership and teamwork: without this the risk exposure and quality of patient care will suffer. Clinical and corporate governance are ways of addressing the quality and risk issues to monitor aspects of integrated care and measure aspects of continuous quality improvements. (These will be discussed further throughout the book.)

THE KEY OBJECTIVES OF THE 1997 WHITE PAPER

The key objectives of the 1997 White Paper are to:

- remove obstacles to integrated care;
- develop services which are responsive to local needs;
- reduce variations in healthcare; and
- work in partnership to provide integrated care.

PRIMARY CARE GROUPS (PCGS)

The 1997 White Paper outlines four levels of PCGs to get primary care services working together to achieve a higher degree of involvement in the commissioning and provision of health and social care services[1]. These levels involve increasing accountability and responsibilities for the PCGs and less control by the health authorities (HAs) whose future role is seen as strategically leading and shaping healthcare with less administrative activities and less bureaucracy. The HAs will lead the developments in the promotion of partnerships and health improvement programmes (HIPs) with the management of local targets and standards, range and location of services, health assessment of needs and the promotion of health across all sectors of health and social care. HAs will work closely with NHS trusts, PCGs, local authorities, academics, public health departments, community health councils, voluntary organisations and the general public. (These will be discussed further in Chapter 5.)

THE FOUR LEVELS OF PCGS

The four levels of PCG activity are as follows.

1. At the minimum level, the PCG will support the health authority in commissioning care for its population, acting in an advisory capacity.
2. At the next level the PCG will take devolved responsibility for managing the budget for healthcare in its area formally as part of the health authority.
3. PCGs can become established as free-standing bodies accountable to the health authority for commissioning care.
4. At the maximum level, the PCGs will become established as free-standing bodies accountable to the health authority for commissioning care and with added responsibility for the provision of community health services for their population.

The PCGs can start at any point on this spectrum and will be expected to develop and move along the levels with increasing accountability and responsibility for local healthcare commissioning, budgetary control, general management, prescribing and integrated care. Some PCGs may choose to stay at levels 1 and 2 without becoming free-standing bodies. It is anticipated that the PCGs will cover populations of around 100 000 and will be responsible for commissioning a comprehensive range of community-based and secondary care hospital services. The proposals mark the end of the internal market and the fragmentation of care. There is no blueprint for what a PCG will look like, what works in one area may not work in another, it has to be horses for courses to account for local needs and health improvements. During 1999, the fund-holding scheme will be wound up and the GP Fundholding Practice Fund Management Allowance of £135m will be redeployed. Extra cash has also been announced by Frank Dobson to set up and develop the PCGs, including extra resources going to non-fundholding practices to restore equity across practices. PCGs will have a budget, which brings together their population's share of hospital and community health services, prescribing, and the general management services (GMS) cash limited budget which in theory should help to promote integrated care in service planning, service development and service delivery in line with local health and social care needs. There is also a need to address health promotion and the prevention of ill-health by using all aspects of integrated care working with public health departments to inform environmental, education, pollution and other social care agencies.

WORKING IN PARTNERSHIP TO PROVIDE INTEGRATED CARE

New statutory duties[1] (subject to legislation) have been imposed on all healthcare providers to participate in the locality health plans and health improvement programmes (HIPs) through consultation, partnership, cooperation, communication and integrated care management[4]. They also have, for the first time, a statutory responsibility (subject to legislation by parliamentary approval) to maintain and improve the quality of care they provide, by processes which are subject to external scrutiny, review and accountability[1]. From April 1999 all healthcare providers will have to guarantee quality of care through a new process called clinical governance. This incorporates a number of processes, including clinical audit; evidence-based practice in daily use supported within the infrastructure; clinical effectiveness; clinical risk management with adverse events being detected, openly investigated and lessons learned; lessons for improving practice being learned from complaints; outcomes of care; good quality clinical data to monitor clinical care with problems of poor clinical practice being recognised early and dealt with; good practice systematically disseminated within and outside the organisation and clinical risk reduction programmes of a high standard being in place. Clinical governance places a duty of responsibility on the chief executive, trust board and all healthcare professionals to ensure that care is 'satisfactory, consistent and responsive: each individual will be responsible for the quality of their clinical practice as part of professional self-regulation'. Every healthcare organisation will need to appoint a doctor, nurse or other clinical professional to take charge of quality issues. There will be a legal duty of quality imposed on every hospital in England for the first time in the history of the NHS[5]. These duties will be subject to external scrutiny, review and accountability. A new organisation, called the Commission for Health Improvement (CHIMP), will be established to police the arrangements for clinical governance in trusts. This organisation will provide external assurance through the implementation of systematic reviews from the national service framework and benchmarking, the NHS charter and national surveys. CHIMP will have wide-ranging powers to inspect trusts, investigate problems, propose changes and recommend action directly to the health secretary. Walshe describes CHIMP as 'a watchdog equipped with both a pleasant smile and sharp teeth'[6].

HEALTHCARE PERFORMANCE MEASUREMENTS

The NHS executive is in the process of setting up a national framework for assessing performance to press for a system based on partnership and driven by performance and to help ensure consistent access to services and quality of care right across the country[7]. The evidence-based national service frameworks will cover major care areas and disease groups to ensure consistency of policy across the NHS. These will be based upon six care areas and 37 high level performance indicators which will assess if the NHS is performing in line with the expectations of the White Paper. There are also indicators in the Green Paper, *Our Healthier Nation*, which include heart disease, cancer, accidents and suicides[8]. The six areas being addressed are: health improvement, fair access, effective delivery of appropriate healthcare, efficiency, patient/carer expectations and health outcome of NHS care.

There will be three new initiatives to support and monitor the NHS changes:

- The NHS Research and Development Programme to assess the clinical and cost-effectiveness of various aspects of healthcare.
- A National Institute of Clinical Excellence (NICE) to promote the use of clinical guidelines derived from evidence-based practice with inbuilt advice on clinical audit criteria and evaluation. It will have a role in the assessment of prime research and systematic reviews and appraisal of clinical guidelines. This new centre will provide information on clinical and cost effectiveness and sharing of best practices.
- The Commission for Health Improvement (CHIMP) will be a statutory body to support those who are developing and monitoring local systems and multidisciplinary standards for clinical quality. It will offer an independent guarantee that local systems to monitor, assure and improve clinical quality are in place. It will also have the capacity to offer specific support on request when local organisations face particular clinical problems. It will also investigate and identify the sources of problems and work with organisations on lasting remedies to improve quality and standards of patient care.

QUALITY OF PATIENT CARE

The NHS reforms have a big impact on the systems for quality of patient care and clinical and organisational risk management and these will be referred to throughout the book. Clinical risk modification should be inherent in the healthcare delivery system and begins with the identification of systems and practices that expose patients to risk of injury, poor quality of care and adverse patient outcomes. The process of risk identification must follow the patient through the delivery system across the sectors of health and social care so that process improvement methods can be broad based for maximum impact.

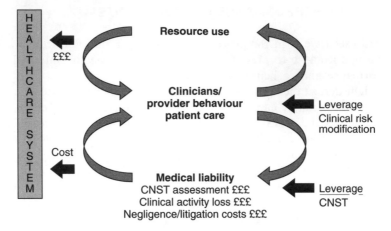

Figure 1.1   Reducing healthcare costs: an integrated systems approach. © 1996, Jo Wilson, HRRI.

After risk exposures have been identified, strategies to improve processes, systems and practices must be defined and implemented. These should be supported and integrated through consultation, information and education but often the hardest part is changing the cultural behaviour and clinical practices. As outlined in Figure 1.1, the best way to reduce costs is to have an integrated system. The resources used and applied to healthcare will never meet the demands which will always outstrip the supply available. There is some leverage by trying to share or pool costs through the Central Negligence Scheme for Trusts (CNST) or transferring the risks for non-clinical care through insurance. (See Chapter 3 for further information.) The best leverage to reduce costs and allow money to be transferred to better higher quality patient care is through clinical risk modification which influences practices, clinical effectiveness and outcomes.

WHITE PAPER AGENDA FOR CHANGE

The programme of change (Figure 1.2) is described as evolutionary over a ten-year period although some primary care team members feel it is more revolutionary and by pushing development too quickly could stifle innovation. The 1997 White Paper sets out the government policy for change in a framework that is permissive in terms of options and details[1]. Many feel things are moving too quickly without clear central guidance leading to local interpretation and trying to be one step ahead. The agenda for change is massive and its success will be determined by the PCGs and how they are allowed to develop and form partnerships with others, in keeping with what has worked well, sharing best practices and allowing local interpretation of the Green Paper *Our Healthier Nation* as a means of 'how to do it'[8]. Healthcare providers

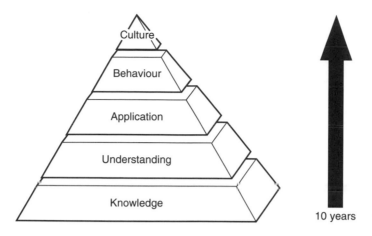

Figure 1.2   Agenda for change in the NHS: evolution not revolution. © 1998, Jo Wilson.

need to discard changes which have resulted in fragmentation, poor coordination and collaboration, unfairness, distortion, inefficiency, instability, secrecy and overburdening due to bureaucracy. PCGs need a period of stability, time to develop, a clear understanding of clinical governance and the framework for performance measurement and quality improvement criteria. This agenda for change needs to be strategically well planned to shift the power base of healthcare delivery and to bring along the key players in all aspects of health and social care to develop their knowledge and understanding, and how they are going to apply the changes to have a successful impact on the behaviour and cultural changes which will influence the radical agenda in the emergence of a new NHS for the 21st century. The action plan must address the following issues to be successful: the pace of change; the appointment process for governing bodies; the further work needed organisation wide; the training and development of PCG governing bodies; and the development of infrastructure to achieve and maintain the changes.

APPROPRIATENESS OF CARE

All three UK White Papers discuss appropriateness of care and how this must become a major focus of quality[1,9,10]. None of the papers gives a clear definition of appropriateness which must be seen as the optimum point of balance between liability and quality as shown in Figure 1.3. This is in line with having the best defensibility in terms of processes and systems if things do go wrong and having the quality assurance standards to demonstrate a controlled environment of care. This must be achieved in line with clinical and cost effectiveness to ensure that we are using our scarce resources to achieve the balance and not practising defensive medicine to cover our backs and for

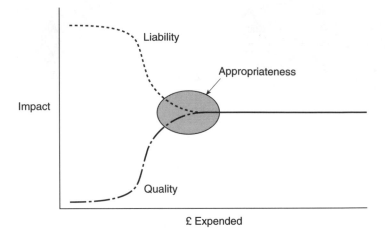

Figure 1.3   A new definition of healthcare risk management. © 1996, Jo Wilson, HRRI.

fear of litigation. The more we spend on quality or defensive medicine, the less effective or appropriate the care becomes in terms of the money spent. The aim should be to move the balance further to the left to spend less and allow appropriateness to become the major focus of quality and liability. However, the preliminary data suggest (Figure 1.4) that quality goes zooming up in one direction to meet patients expectations and appropriateness declines in the opposite direction as it is not clearly defined and accepted[4]. We do need to get these more in balance in line with evidence-based research/practice and clinical effectiveness.

The NHS White Paper certainly sets the agenda for evolutionary change with everyone taking a responsibility for improving quality and getting it right first time and every time. To achieve this balance appropriateness must

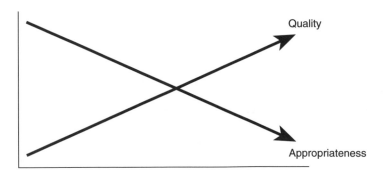

Figure 1.4   Relationship between quality and appropriateness suggested by preliminary data. © 1996, Jo Wilson, HRRI.

become the major focus for quality and it is not just how well you do it but whether activities/procedures should be done in the first place. To achieve this balance there needs to be better understanding of the synergy between clinical risk/governance, quality and the legal issues to achieve true clinical risk modification to change practice, behaviour and eventually the culture of the NHS and its practitioners. Quality of care is everyone's business and we need to demonstrate this to the public to restore their faith in our healthcare delivery systems.

Patients also must have more responsibility for their healthcare. They should be accountable for keeping appointments, making better use of facilities, and efficient use of NHS resources. Today healthcare professionals practise in an environment with increasing patient expectations, seeing the NHS as similar to the commercial world. Within the NHS there is a trend towards patients resorting to litigation and to making formal complaints. If patients get an unexpected outcome or have not been appropriately communicated with or have not given true informed consent, they are more likely to take action to receive better information or seek some form of compensation.

CLINICAL RISK MODIFICATION

In this environment a knowledge of the law and the legal system becomes an essential prerequisite for reflective professional practice. It is clearly important to try to understand trends and why patients sue and complain and to adjust professional practice accordingly.

This book attempts to provide an overview and insights into the changes in the NHS and their impact on the risk modification agenda and the importance of clinical and corporate governance. Included are the main principles of clinical risk management, cultural and behaviour changes and discussions about some main legal principles. Reasons why patients sue and complain are very important to us as practitioners and these are also discussed.

Two legal chapters have been included to illustrate the relevance and application of the law to healthcare practice and to clinical risk management. The legal principles discussed include those relating to consent to treatment and medical negligence. A good clinical risk modification strategy should comply with the law.

THE LITIGATION SPIRAL

The levels and costs of healthcare litigation are high and rising fast as Department of Health figures show[11].

> The total cost of NHS clinical negligence litigation is currently estimated at around £200 million, and is likely to grow at nearly 25 per cent per annum

over the next five years, of which the share directly borne by trusts will rise from about 10 per cent to 75 per cent.

Latest figures show a record increase to £300 million in 1996–7[12]. The DOH estimates[13] that the cost of clinical negligence claims in the year 2000–1 will be around £500m. Projections are inevitably uncertain but a general pattern can be seen.

The increasing cost of litigation is seen as a reflection of[13]:

1. increases in the volume of NHS activity;
2. the increasing tendency for patients to seek redress when incidents occur; and
3. continuing upward pressures on the size of negligence awards over and above the general level of litigation.

The DOH suggests that trusts can take a number of steps to mitigate these increasing costs[13]. Trusts can:

● adopt prudent risk management strategies;
● implement in full the new complaints procedure;
● adopt a systematic approach to claims handling in line with current best practice and in accordance with advice issued by the NHSLA (National Health Service Litigation Authority); and
● consider joining the CNST (Clinical Negligence Scheme for Trusts).

The NHSLA and CNST are discussed in Chapter 3; they are clearly an important feature of the clinical risk modification environment and have an important impact on claims handling procedures.

A COMPLAINTS SPIRAL?

The new complaints systems in healthcare are discussed in Chapters 6 and 7. Complaints also show an increase. The HSC (Health Service Commissioner or Ombudsman) Michael Buckley in his first annual report as HSC received 2219 complaints about the NHS, 24 per cent up on the previous year and an all-time record[14]. In 1996–97 the HSC upheld 93 per cent of all complaints to the HSC about complaint-handling by health authorities or trusts, compared with 65 per cent in 1989–90 and 90 per cent in 1996.

A complainant can easily turn into a litigant and the importance of good complaint handling cannot be stressed strongly enough. Effective strategies are discussed in Chapter 7.

WHY DO PATIENTS SUE AND COMPLAIN?

It is the experience of many healthcare professionals and lawyers that many patients complain and sue out of a feeling of frustration. If they cannot obtain a proper explanation for the untoward incident that has happened to them or a relative, complaining and going to a solicitor are the last resorts. Experience suggests that communication problems are behind most complaints (as discussed in Chapter 2) and a good number of court cases. If patient and healthcarer communication strategies are improved there will be a demonstrable decrease in litigation and complaint levels.

Vincent, Young and Phillips' study supports this view[15]. They examined the reasons why patients and their relatives take legal action. They surveyed 227 patients and relatives who were taking legal action through five firms of plaintiff medical negligence solicitors. They found that the decision to take legal action was determined not only by the original injury, but also by insensitive handling and poor communication after the original incident. Where explanations were given, less than 15 per cent were considered satisfactory.

AVMA (Action for Victims of Medical Accidents) maintains a similar view and states that the vast majority of patients who have experienced something going wrong during medical care, or their relatives if the patient has died, are not interested in compensation[16]. Money, they say, cannot compensate for the loss of a child or another loved one or for the loss of health.

> What they want is 'satisfaction'. What that means is a full explanation of what went wrong, an honest explanation of why it went wrong and, if appropriate, an apology for what actually happened. They will also want to be assured that all steps will be taken to ensure that a similar accident does not happen to someone else in the future. Of course, there are times when financial compensation is also necessary and that will form part of the 'satisfaction' that the patient wants.

Effective communication strategies should, as a matter of practical necessity, underpin all clinical risk management strategies.

CHANGES IN THE LITIGATION PROCESS

Cheryl Blundell, in her chapter, discusses the future of medical litigation in the light of the Woolf reforms. Change in the litigation system is inevitable and reform is much needed. It is important at the beginning of a text that looks at clinical risk modification to remind ourselves why Lord Woolf looked at medical negligence and the problems he found, as they provide a useful focus and perspective for debate[17].

> . . . early in the Inquiry it became increasingly obvious that it was in the area of medical negligence that the civil justice system was failing most conspicuously to meet the needs of litigants in a number of respects.
>
> 1. The disproportion between costs and damages in medical negligence is particularly excessive, especially in lower value cases.
> 2. The delay in resolving claims is more often unacceptable.

3. Unmeritorious cases are often pursued, and clear-cut claims defended for too long.
4. The success rate is lower than in other personal injury litigation.
5. The suspicion between the parties is more intense and the lack of co-operation frequently greater than in many other areas of litigation.

These points raised by the Woolf report and his recommendations for reform create an important reform agenda.

REFERENCES

1. Department of Health (1997) *The New NHS, Modern, Dependable.* Cmnd 3807. HMSO Office: London.
2. Department of Health (1989) *Working for Patients.* HMSO: London.
3. Department of Health (1996) *Choice and Opportunity, Primary Care: The Future.* Cmnd 3390. HMSO: London.
4. Wilson, J. H. (1996) *Integrated Care Management: The Path to Success.* Butterworth-Heinemann: Oxford.
5. Department of Health (1998) Press Release 98/141, 13 April 1998. *NHS to have a legal duty of ensuring quality for the first time.* DOH: London.
6. Walshe, K. (1998) Cutting to the heart of quality. *Health Management,* **May,** 20–21.
7. NHS Executive (1998) *The New NHS, Modern, and Dependable: A National Framework for Assessing Performance.* 12394 FPA 5k 2P Feb 98 (RIC). HMSO: London.
8. Department of Health (1998) *Our Healthier Nation.* CM3852. HMSO: London.
9. The Scottish Office Department of Health (1997) *Designed to Care.* Cmnd 3811. The Stationery Office: Edinburgh.
10. The Welsh Office Department of Health (1997) *Putting Patients First.* HMSO: London.
11. Department of Health (1996) *Clinical Negligence and Personal Injury Litigation: Claims Handling.* EL(96)11. NHS Executive, DOH: Leeds.
12. Hansard (1998) House of Commons debate for 24 March, column 165. HMSO: London.
13. Department of Health (1996) *Clinical Negligence Costs.* FDL (96)39, October. NHS Executive, DOH: Leeds.
14. HSC (1998) *First Report for Session 1997–98, Annual Report for 1996–97.* HMSO: London.
15. Vincent, C., Young, M. and Phillips, A. (1994) Why do people sue doctors? A study of patients and relatives taking legal action. *The Lancet,* **343,** 1609–1613.
16. Action for Victims of Medical Accidents (1995) *Medical Accidents.* AVMA: London.
17. Lord Woolf (1996) *Access to Justice: Final Report.* HMSO: London.

2 APPLYING CLINICAL RISK MODIFICATION IN PRACTICE

Jo Wilson

INTRODUCTION

Clinical risk modification provides the best service for patients through obtaining a synergy between risk management, quality and the law. It also allows for the establishment of multidisciplinary standards of care and best-practice guidelines to enhance professional development of nursing, therapy professions and medicine. The changes in healthcare delivery, with much higher expectations from patients, greater clarity of roles and responsibilities of clinicians and the emphasis on devolving decision making as close to the patient as possible, is meant to affect the entire performance of healthcare delivery. For most senior managers, nurses and doctors, the environment in which they operate has grown increasingly turbulent and complex with increasing demands on resources and increases in workload. They must contend with the more universal issues of monitoring patient activity, quality and evaluation through clinical audit, cost control, providing accessible and equitable services with relevance to the local population healthcare needs and social acceptability, as well as efficiency and effectiveness – all while ensuring their organisations' survival.

The commissioners of healthcare, on behalf of their clients, look for the best and most efficient healthcare delivery systems giving the best value for money by improving access, equity and quality of care without increasing the cost of services. To improve value, providers must understand and maximise the linkages between its two basic components – cost and quality. Both the cost and quality of care are components in determining the value of the healthcare delivered, and both are elements of healthcare risk. To begin to manage these elements of risk, the process of healthcare risk modification can be applied. The focus of healthcare risk modification is intensely on the systems and practices that affect patient care in order proactively to manage overall cost and appropriateness of care delivered. All aspects of the system – physical works, equipment, security, training, management, nursing, medicine, allied health professionals, etc. – have a role and responsibilities in increasing or modifying healthcare risk.

TOOLS OF RISK MODIFICATION

The tools of risk modification are designed to be proactive and to concentrate on helping the multidisciplinary team to minimise and/or eliminate the cause of the identified potential risk. They should be used to assist professionals in the audit and evaluation of their healthcare delivery with local ownership and control. They also serve as a change management mechanism for the healthcare organisation striving towards the best outcomes. This approach requires clear mechanisms for risk prone areas:

- For dealing with emergencies, staff awareness and understanding of clear trauma and major accident (MAJAX) plans should be tested by regular drills.
- Service level agreements with quality criteria, which are subject to regular audit, are required for clinical supporting services such as radiology, social work, social services, laboratory services, community care and operating theatres.
- Patients' and children's charters should define clear expectations of service delivery including waiting times and of what is required from patients for efficient and effective care delivery.
- For the organisational risks there should be contingency and disaster recovery plans for the management of potential crises involving for example fire, explosions, lapses of security, water pollution/failures, breakdowns of air conditioning, piped medical gas failures, sewage contamination, breaches or failures of power, telecommunications, information technology, building, plant and equipment, disposal of waste and infection control systems.

The tools for risk identification are summarised in Table 2.1 and these will be explained throughout the text to enhance the understanding of clinical risk modification.

Table 2.1 Risk identification tools © 1994, Jo Wilson, HRRI

☐ Incident reports	☐ Contract information/service quality level agreements
☐ Clinical audit/effectiveness/quality criteria	☐ Survey reports
☐ Committee reports and minutes	☐ Clinical indicators
☐ Claims data	☐ Patient records review/documentation of care
☐ Patient complaints	☐ Channels of communication
☐ Policies and procedures	

RISK

Risk in its simplest form is the potential for unwanted outcome[1]. This is a very broad definition which includes patient dissatisfaction from having to wait too long or not being communicated with, to the patient having the wrong operation or suffering permanent disability or wrongful death. The concept of risk can be defined in an English dictionary as 'chance or possibility of loss or bad consequence'[2]; in an American dictionary as 'exposure to the chance of injury or loss; hazard or dangerous chance'[3]. Williams and Heins define risk as 'a variation in the outcomes that could occur over a specified period in a given situation'[4]. While the dictionary definitions are more general, the Williams and Heins definition provides a clearer understanding of the application of the concept. This can be further applied to healthcare settings where risk takes several forms:

- Patient injury while in the healthcare organisation's care results in extensive resource utilisation to correct the injury.
- Decreased productivity results from time and resources spent in clinical negligence litigation.
- The reputation of the healthcare provider is adversely affected by patient injury incidents.
- There may be clinical liability awards to injured parties and legal costs related to the litigation process.
- Patient unhappiness and dissatisfaction is often due to lack of information and ineffective communication.
- There are hidden costs in terms of pain and injury, locum cover costs, stress suffered by the individuals involved and reduction in the quality of care delivery. There are resource costs of replacement, facility downtime and service improvements. Also the risk of the tarnishing of the reputations of the professionals involved and the profile of the organisation. Added to this is the cost of public relations and crisis management to improve local and public perceptions of the healthcare facility and its staff and services.

In each of these we can see elements of financial costs and decreased quality which can place providers at a distinct disadvantage within the healthcare system.

RISK MODIFICATION

Modification is the changing of circumstances, the environment and behaviour ultimately to lower the potential for and amount of healthcare risk. The risk management tools help to identify areas where healthcare continuous quality improvements can be made. The result is improved outcomes, patient satisfaction and the documentation of care delivery. Poor communication between professionals and with patients is the most common reason for patients/

relatives to make complaints or even take out litigation to acquire the necessary explanation and information. The Medical Protection Society estimates that in 90 per cent of cases presented to it over a three year period, failure to communicate featured as a major component of the case. In addition, Action for Victims of Medical Accidents (AVMA) estimates that more than 50 per cent of the complaints it receives are due to communication problems. To modify clinical risk and manage it appropriately our two best forms of risk prevention are effective communication and excellent documentation. This chapter will concentrate on developing these risk prevention tools to demonstrate ways of showing how effective they can be.

Management is designing and directing activities that establish the conditions for organisation success within the context of service delivery. Management should evaluate the effectiveness of clinical practice, patient satisfaction and outcomes, and examine the frequency/severity and defensibility of claims. This does not mean practising defensive medicine but having the best defensibility in place if and when things do go wrong.

Taken together, these definitions create a broader interpretation of risk management and begin to present risk solutions – through the implementation of risk modification for providers of healthcare.

Risk management is the systematic identification, assessment and reduction of risks to patients and staff:

- through providing appropriate, effective and efficient levels of patient care;
- by prevention and avoidance of untoward incidents and events;
- by learning lessons and changing behaviour/practices as a result of near misses, incidents and adverse outcomes; and
- through communication and documentation of care in a comprehensive, objective, consistent and accurate way.

CLINICAL NEGLIGENCE

Litigation for clinical negligence has been rising dramatically in recent years (as we saw in Chapter 1). The NHS Management Executive[5] has quoted some recent costs to the NHS which have risen from £53m in 1990/1 to £125m in 1993/4, £150m in 1994/5, £200m in 1995/6 and an estimated £250m in 1996/7. One way of reducing this is through clinical risk modification by proactively managing the systems and practices that affect patient care, including effective communication, documentation and integrated care, and thereby reducing subsequent litigation through claims management. A Clinical Negligence Scheme for Trusts (CNST) has been set up in England as a mutual pooling arrangement; similarly there is the Welsh Risk Pool (WRP) for Wales (for further details on the CNST and WRP see Chapter 3).

The CNST/WRP are voluntary schemes enabling healthcare organisations and health authorities to pool the cost of clinical negligence settlements each year in return for an annual subscription, bearing in mind that (in the final analysis) prevention is cheaper than cure. They are designed to assist the NHS trust to meet the cost of clinical negligence claims, to promote effective risk and claim management and improve the cost and quality of service delivery.

The emphasis is on the adoption of prudent risk management strategies; meeting the CNST and WRP risk management standards; implementing in full the new complaints procedure including its potential linkages to near misses, clinical indicators and clinical incidents to provide an alternative remedy for some potential litigants and adopting a systematic approach to claims handling in line with best practice. The risk management standards are focused upon the organisational, communication and documentation issues, which are all inter-related to the prevention and minimisation of risk exposure. A clear chain of command with individual roles and responsibilities ensures that risks are managed and reflects the commitment of the trust board members. This ensures that policies, procedures and clinical guidelines are updated to maintain safe systems of work for patients, staff and visitors. Staff are orientated and inducted appropriately to the organisation at trust and specialty levels and this also refers to locums, bank and agency staff. Informed consent receives a high weighting at all levels with an increased need for providing information leaflets and communicating with patients the risks, alternatives and benefits of all invasive procedures.

TOOLS OF RISK IDENTIFICATION

Incident reporting

Risk management is a process for the identification of risks which have adverse effects on the quality, safety and effectiveness of service delivery; the assessment and evaluation of those risks; and positive action to eliminate or reduce them. Having an open, honest and blame-free organisation which is open to improving processes and systems of care is a big step towards having staff committed to quality and getting things right. Near-miss, incident and indicator recording and reporting are a cornerstone of any quality and risk management system.

Incident reporting, investigation and follow-up are considered a minimum, level one, standard of the Clinical Negligence Scheme for Trusts, alongside the clinical complaints procedure as a means of assessing areas where improvements need to be made[6]. The reporting of near misses is also important as we can learn from these and put systems in place to stop them happening. These will be discussed in more details in Chapters 3 and 4. Risk reduction will also flow from a positive approach to risk containment and control. It is important to turn what appear to be overwhelming difficulties into opportunities for improvement. Every near miss, complaint and incident which is reported presents a chance to learn from past errors to improve the services in the future.

Clinical audit, effectiveness and quality criteria

These need to work in harmony with risk management allowing each to inform the other and allow for true clinical effectiveness and the development of evidence-based practice. Risk and quality are two sides of the same coin; experience has shown where there is good quality there is low risk and there is a strong synergy between them. Many healthcare organisations now have a clinical effectiveness department which allows the criteria and results to work together. Risk can highlight areas for further audit, quality deficiencies can be identified from an audit review and risk assessments can inform the ongoing audit process. These elements will be discussed further and applied throughout the book.

Committee reports and minutes

Committee structure and output play a key role in risk management and clinical effectiveness in terms of recording decision making and changes in policies and practices. It is important that this is a two-way process with information and decisions influencing healthcare changes and controlling risk modification. The organisation's risk management strategy should clearly identify the roles and responsibilities of committees and who needs to action certain information. There need to be clear reporting, review and evaluation processes which can be demonstrated within the minutes, including decisions to change systems and practices.

Claims management

The cost of claims for clinical negligence continues to rise rapidly. To protect your organisation and its people it is essential to have a comprehensive and focused claims management programme.

The organisation needs to develop skills in the following areas:

- comprehensive administration of claims;
- early identification of claims through complaints and incident tracking;
- evaluation, assessment and reserving of claims,
- full investigation of events including reports and statements;
- disposition by direct negotiation or other forms of dispute resolution, loss and reserve tracking; and
- services which are designed to work with their data management systems.

All skills should be supported by compatible data management including complaint, incident and claim tracking and clinical evaluation systems. This includes fulfilling the reporting requirements of all bodies responsible for funding the litigation.

Claims management systems development

Organisations are starting to review their information and communication systems to ensure that they make their claims management process a success by having in place an infrastructure to address cost, risk efforts and clinical outcomes. This will include:

- the integration and information sharing processes of risk, quality/audit and claims;
- enhancing the organisation's requirements and education programme;
- developing your current systems or assisting you in procuring a claims information system best suited to your requirements;
- the expertise to develop a system tailored specifically to your organisation; and
- the stages of reporting requirements for claims including the sharing of information and confidentiality issues.

Claims file review

On a regular basis there needs to be a file review to ensure that all open files are monitored closely according to your organisation's requirements.

Comprehensive ongoing reviews should:

- review all your open and on-going claims to ensure that they are progressing in the organisation's best interests;
- recommend actions to monitor the litigation process as well as advising on settlement to achieve expedited resolution of claims, thereby reducing unnecessary legal costs; and
- produce a report identifying the file defence strategy.

Periodically auditing your claims handling process should include:

- a review of a sample of both open and closed claims to ensure that they are being well managed and adequately resolved; and
- the provision of a detailed report of findings with recommendations to improve your organisation's claims management and reduce legal costs.

Legal advice from organisation solicitors

It is essential for the organisation to be provided with the best and most cost-effective support from external legal advisers.

- They should conduct an audit to ensure that external claims management (product, employee, clinical and public liability) legal services provided to the organisation are of an acceptable quality.
- They should also develop expertise in assisting your organisation in the procurement of external legal services as is appropriate.

Education and training

The organisation should be provided with ongoing education and training in the following areas:

- participation training workshops for managers and clinicians in the principles of risk and claims management;
- focused training workshops to identified individuals involved specifically with the risk and claims management functions; and
- mentored one-to-one claims management training working alongside an identified person to facilitate skills transfer and knowledge of the process.

Patient complaints

Communication and lack of information are two major issues which cause significant problems for healthcare organisations. These issues often come to light in the form of patient complaints which may be viewed negatively by the organisation. They need to be viewed much more positively. They are 'jewels', 'free lessons' or free market research where customers tell us what they are not satisfied with or where improvements can be made. Many organisations take the '3Cs' approach: this involves monitoring comments, compliments and complaints and using their ratios to manage service improvements. For these reasons it is important to mention complaints in this chapter but they will be covered in much further detail in Chapters 4, 7 and 8. Complaints should be linked into incident reporting, claims management and access to patient records requests to ensure early identification of potential clinical negligence.

There is a definite increase in the number of complaints in the NHS correlated with rising patient expectations of healthcare delivery. This increase is demonstrated by the Health Service Commissioner's Reports which showed: in 1992 a 4 per cent increase in the number of complaints to 1227, a further increase in 1993/4 of 12.8 per cent to 1384, in 1994/5 increases of 25 per cent, and in 1996/7 a record number of 2219 complaints, 24 per cent up on the previous year[7]. In addition, the Commissioner processed 2207 items of supplementary correspondence, an increase of 30 per cent. The reports state[7]:

> There are some awful examples in the report of delay, incomplete or incomprehensible replies, lack of sensitivity, victimisation and refusal to permit the presence of a friend at a complaint discussion.

In April 1996 the Health Service Commissioner's remit changed to include investigations into clinical complaints and the same recurring themes have continued: failures by staff to communicate with each other, poor record keeping and failures in administration or communication at the time of a patient's death which compound the grief of relatives. Failure to communicate is again stated to be the central reason for complaints. Patients view the NHS in the same light as they view other services and there is a greater call for accountability in healthcare provision. Good communication and documentation is fundamental to effective clinical practice. The best way to support these elements is through good contemporary record keeping ensuring that appropriate information is recorded. If things are not written down it is hard to find proof that they did happen in accordance with the verbal report and it can often result in one person's word against another.

Policies and procedures

The importance of up-to-date, easily understood clinical policies, procedures, guidelines, treatment protocols and agreed standards cannot be over-emphasised in relation to risk reduction. Often, a major cause of risk is that members of staff are individually uncertain of what is expected of them, particularly in emergency situations. This can be compounded when other members of the same team have different understandings about what actions should be taken in such circumstances.

The organisation should ensure that policies and procedures are up-to-date; issued to those who need to use them; received and read by those people; understood by those people, and put into action by those people. Furthermore, regular audits should be undertaken to ensure staff awareness and compliance with them, within clear lines of accountability.

The organisation should have a continuous programme for reviewing all of the hospital's policies and procedures, protocols, pathways and guidelines to ensure that they are clear, concise, dated and updated annually. Medical, nursing and other procedures will be research-based, and procedure manuals and documents will include a reference section. Too many policies, procedures and guidelines can be as risky as having none if they contradict and confuse staff due to overlap and inconsistency. It is better to have fewer relevant guidelines than hundreds which only serve to confuse staff who find there are so many they do not bother or cannot find the time to read them.

The organisation should also ensure that the organisation-wide policies, procedures, guidelines and pathways are sufficiently flexible to be of practical use in different services and departments, without leading to inconsistency in interpretation. Accordingly, all policies will make clear what must be strictly followed, and what is open to managerial discretion. A clear framework needs to be set up for monitoring compliance and non-compliance with the ordinances using the roles of the subject officers to determine the criteria and perform the ongoing observation, measurement, monitoring and evaluation. Consistency in the management and retention of obsolete or superseded documents should be developed to ensure that there is always a core set kept for reference.

Contract information and service quality level agreements

To maximise patient safety and continuity of care it is recommended that service level agreements are set up with clear quality criteria and acceptable standards which can be measured and audited. These should include all internal contracts and agreements internally between specialties and support departments and externally with other agencies and service providers. There has to be an appreciation of the different pressures on staff groups within their own working environment to meet realistic expectations. Undertaking reviews by responding to crises and non-delivery of expectations is unrealistic and amounts to fire fighting. Service level quality agreements support proactive management by measuring and monitoring the service provided in the best interest of the patient.

Survey reports

Surveys undertaken by external organisations in the form of accreditation, organisational audits, risk reviews and audit commission reports should be used proactively to achieve continuous quality improvements and modify risk management practices. These are usually objective reports by people who can come into your organisation as 'a fresh pair of eyes and ears' and can highlight positive practices and areas for improvements. Sometimes these reports are accepted and even action planning takes place, but often they lose direction within the organisation. These reports should be used to inform the quality, audit, risk and clinical effectiveness agendas. The organisation needs to take ownership and control so that it can utilise the information to the best advantage.

Clinical indicators

Clinically focused indicators based upon claims analysis serve as triggers or early warning signs for issues which have the potential for things to go wrong if appropriate action is not taken. They are usually determined by national task forces of experts and they contribute to the effective management of liability risk. Indicators raise awareness among all providers of systems and practices which can lead to untoward patient outcomes and increased morbidity, mortality and cost per case. They provide 'top of the tree' triggers or early warning signs which look at events that serve as a flag for deeper review, timely comparative data source with potential benchmarking opportunities and the provision of drivers for decision making and the promotion of behaviour changes. These will be discussed further with examples in Chapters 3 and 4.

Patient records

Proactive clinical risk management addresses the identification of existing risks, the assessment of potential system failures, the analysis of priorities for action and the elimination or reduction of potential or actual hazards. One of the ways of starting to review and be more preventative is by addressing the issues of clinical effectiveness, evidenced-based practice and better utilisation of clinical outcomes. Clinical effectiveness, quality, audit and risk management can be brought together under one umbrella to outline clear processes and systems of healthcare delivery. This can be undertaken by addressing the following matters.

- The systematic monitoring of quality and appropriateness of patient care.
- The identification of deviations from standards of care, evidence-based practice, patient injuries or other situations that reflect exposure.
- The modification of high-risk practices.
- The establishment and use of agreed clinical guidelines and Multidisciplinary Pathways of Care[©8].

There are two important components of healthcare which regularly let practitioners down and are also two of the best methods of risk prevention. These are the documentation and the communication of the care delivery processes. This chapter will start to identify the issues around the documentation of care and some of the communication issues.

Staff need to be more aware and involved in the audit and evaluation of documentation of care and should regularly undertake reviews of their patients' records.

The Audit Commission's reports on the examination of patient records confirms the Health Service Commissioner's view of record keeping in nursing as ritualistic and lacking essential information[9].

The problems found with patient records were the following:

- records undated and unsigned,
- lack of detail about the person rather than the medical problem;
- insufficient information about the patient's perception of the problem and response to treatment;
- patient's psychological and emotional needs not documented;
- objectives for care not established;
- progress towards care objectives not evaluated; and
- assessments for discharge and discharge plans not documented.

Clinicians are reminded that accurate record keeping and documentation with regular quality review and audit is essential. Tracking patients and their care throughout the healthcare organisation can only be achieved by checking patient identity and making adequate patient record entries. A comprehensive, objective, accurate, complete and consistent record of patient care in the patient record is the best defence if anything untoward does happen.

Where do the common pitfalls occur?
The most common problems with patient records include the following.

- Lack of clear policies, procedures and clinical guidelines.
- Insufficient care and attention given to the informed consent process and the communication and discussion of the risks, alternatives and benefits of the proposed treatments.
- Conflicting information providing an unclear picture and inconsistent record of events.
- Non-standard abbreviations and comments, e.g. FLK (funny looking kid), TATSP (thick as two short planks), PITA (pain in the ass), this patient resembles an orthopaedic museum.
- Subjectivity: document facts, not opinions.
- Preservation of documents in terms of efficient storage, easy and speedy retrieval and complete retention.
- Issues of timing and contemporary recording and not adding entries after the event without adequate explanation, date, time and signature.
- Corrections and spacing: staff continue to obliterate by crossing out or using liquid paper or even adding entries out of sequence without the date, time and reasons.
- Record all significant events: lack of clinical audit of patient records.
- Medication recording is one of the big problems in terms of being able to read the script, the route, the amount, the time of administration and the associated signatures.
- Documented conflict between the professional groups.
- Remember that if it is not in the record, it did not happen.

Review of patient-related documents
Patient-related documents should be reviewed by asking the following questions.

- Is it timely? Delays cause sketchy records and inaccuracies: avoid speculation about the patient's condition.
- Is it objective? Describe assessment or events, avoid frivolous statements and criticisms of care.
- Is it process orientated? For example: are interventions followed by the patient's response? Can the care be compared to your interdisciplinary standards?
- Does it include reassuring information, supported by reference to clinical guidelines and patient information leaflets?
- Is the entire record retrievable and legible? The idea of the record is to share the plan of care with all staff to enhance patient safety and quality of care.
- Are there alterations, use of liquid paper or use of inappropriate terms such as 'the baby was flat and blue'?

Quality assurance activities should include a review of the following areas to address risk issues in the patient's record:

- legibility;
- use of approved abbreviations only;
- use of a signature bank to maintain a record of signatures and printed names;
- completion of all areas of the patient's documents;
- healthcare practitioners' identification by name and title and, in the case of junior doctors, the name of the consultant for whom they are working;
- evidence of dating and timing of all patient record entries;
- objective documentation of patient complaints and response to treatment with tracking and trending in report format;
- evidence of discharge instructions from the clinic, ward or department and the information provided to the patient;
- evidence of documentation of patient teaching and preparation for theatre or procedures and family interaction;
- completed and consistent documentation of multidisciplinary care through-out the patient's full span of care within the healthcare organisation.

The healthcare provider should be able to show demonstrable results in risk reduction from the clinical audit process. The clinical audit process should be developed by a multidisciplinary team and should include, but not be limited to, the following:

- clinically valid standards of care set by the team and incorporated into the healthcare organisation documentation, patient waiting times, and the giving and recording of telephone advice;
- agreed standards of care set by the multidisciplinary team linked to Multi-disciplinary Pathways of Care[©8], protocols, policies and practice guidelines;
- specific thresholds used to monitor compliance with established standards, clinical guidelines and evidence-based practice;
- defined methods for the collection and analysis of data, including reference to collection tools, sample size, time frame and staff responsibility;
- provisions for corrective action planning to include education oppor-tunities, organisational modifications and behavioural changes;
- evidence of follow-up assessment to evaluate the effectiveness of the correc-tive action and ongoing results;
- recognition and maintenance of good practices.

Evaluation of patient care should include, but not be limited to, the following:

- completeness and legibility of patient records, care plans, informed consent and investigation results;
- accuracy of diagnosis, operations/procedures, treatment and follow-on care including allergies and the care delivery processes;

- appropriateness of laboratory investigations, routine radiology procedures and other services;
- the safe and secure movement of patients through the healthcare organisation and the recording of information communicated between staff;
- outcome of care in the short, medium and long term;
- review of patients who leave before examination, and those who discharge against medical advice;
- review of patients with a mental health history and those intoxicated on arrival at the healthcare organisation.

The goals of risk prevention in aspects of record keeping are:

- to provide and document maximum quality of care;
- to recognise and document clearly events that may provide exposure;
- to implement and record measures to reduce exposure; and
- to monitor and record outcomes to ensure quality of patient care.

Successful risk management is becoming less of a matter of procedures, and more a matter of *teamwork* that manages the care and documents the processes appropriately no matter where the healthcare delivery takes place. Working in teams also requires an effective two-way process of sharing of information and communication.

Communication

Communication is the most powerful tool in clinical practice and repeatedly research has shown that good communication skills result in better clinical outcomes, greater propensity to follow clinical recommendations and reduced risk of clinical negligence and complaints. A study by Lester and Smith demonstrated that time-limited, negative communication by doctors is associated with increased litigious intentions among patients, even when outcomes were neither adverse nor negligent[10]. The qualities of caring and concern exhibited by doctors make a difference in healthcare outcomes.

There are three main qualities which are essential to good clinical practice:

- *integrity* – the personal commitment to be honest and trustworthy in evaluating and demonstrating one's own skills and abilities;
- *respect* – the personal commitment to honour others' choices and rights in clinical care; and
- *compassion* – an appreciation that suffering and illness engender special needs for comfort and help.

A number of researchers have shown that these caring qualities can be associated with desired clinical outcomes. Engel said[11]:

> . . . the interview is the most powerful, encompassing and sensitive instrument available to the physician.

His view was that caring and compassionate communication between clinicians and patients is both a central task and at the heart of clinical care delivery. Yet research by Beckman and Frankel showed that[12]:

> Patients have, on average, 18 s to tell their concerns to a physician before being interrupted. Once interrupted, they are unlikely to raise additional concerns before the end of the visit, where such concerns are unlikely to be addressed thoroughly or completely.

Many problems arise from pressure due to working conditions such as time pressures, interruptions and missing or incomplete patient records. Yet we know that employing such skills does not add substantially to the length of visits and can reduce the risk of complaints and clinical negligence claims.

Distressing and challenging as the task of communicating bad news can be, it also represents a significant opportunity for clinicians to influence the process of care positively. Far from an admission of defeat, communicating bad news often is the first step in the development of deeper, more meaningful and satisfying relationships with patients and families. The use of empathy and its associated skills in building therapeutic relationships has been shown to have a strong positive influence on patient satisfaction and compliance. It is important to distinguish empathy from sympathy. Empathy involves recognition and reflection of the patient's feelings, whereas sympathy has the opposite effect and is a more directly parallel response to emotion. Combining empathy and sympathy gives the clinician a broad range of legitimate responses to patients' expressions of negative and painful feelings and can reduce anxiety in the clinician.

Pitfalls of poor communication

Many clinicians, regardless of their training, tend to lack effective communication skills when giving information about diagnosis, prognosis and treatment. Many of these poor communication skills are due to the following:

- failure to notice when the patient is not taking in or accepting the information being offered;
- shrinking from explaining uncomfortable topics;
- failure to appreciate the importance the patient places on receiving appropriate information;
- the perception gap between the patient and clinician, for example the undemanding patient may still wish to be fully informed;
- fear of litigation, especially about how much information to give, and fears regarding discussions of possible risks, alternatives, benefits and hazards of treatments.

The integrated care management process has been able to show vast improvements in the gathering of data, developing relationships and communicating information to and involving patients and other clinicians in partnership for high-quality care delivery[13].

Best practice for communication with patients
Best practice has the following features.

- Listen carefully to what the patient tells you.
- Make sure the patient understands what you say, and reinforce with good, clear information leaflets.
- Do not talk down to the patient or be condescending, but take time to answer questions.
- Avoid inadvertent or unintentional communication.
- Avoid frivolous or critical statements about colleagues.
- Keep the patient fully informed and part of the decision making.
- Respect the patient's wishes and avoid negative verbal or non-verbal cues.

Information should be given to patients in as calm an environment as possible, where time can be spent explaining and answering questions. Too often patients are afraid to ask because they are aware that staff are busy, other patients are waiting and they are very respectful of the clinician's expertise – 'the doctor knows best'. Often patients are anxious about their illness and its consequences which can make it difficult to concentrate on the information being given and the shock of hearing the news or diagnosis can mean the patient not remembering what has been said. Information should be supported by 'plain English' easily understood information leaflets with diagrams, which should also be produced in different languages and with pictures for children.

Best practice for communication with colleagues
Best practice includes the following:

- clear guidelines and clinical management plans;
- clear criteria and shared patient management plans for high-risk cases;
- sharing and passing on information within the team;
- open systems for juniors to seek help and opinions;
- adequate clinical records and communication of care;
- good team work and respect for team members; and
- sharing of communication and documentation with appropriate health and social care organisations.

INTEGRATED CARE MANAGEMENT

As stated above effective communication and excellent documentation of patient care can be addressed through the process of integrated care management (ICM). Over the past few years there have been a number of initiatives which have addressed the importance of patient centred care based upon the appropriateness of, and need for, quick, collaborative, coordinated and reliable service delivery. Integrated care management is at the leading edge of these initiatives as it sets out to address quality criteria in terms of clinical effectiveness and evidence-based practice[13]. Quality criteria are used to inform, provide and make the best decisions possible, which are responsive to the needs and wishes of patients and carers. ICM is a system used to improve the usage of scarce resources by providing the right care to the right patient, in the right place at the right time and for the right reasons by the right people, in a seamless, cost and clinically effective and evidence-based way. Managing healthcare effectively depends significantly upon close monitoring, communication and documentation of patient and family needs throughout the continuum of care. The quality standards, ongoing monitoring and patient outcomes of treatment and care should be the same no matter where the care is provided. The more efficiently this is done, the more the healthcare provider's resources and risk management can be promptly integrated into a flow of interventions which benefit, educate and inform patients. ICM (Table 2.2) can also aid professional development, promote multiprofessional and team working, and provide the context for ongoing training and development.

The recent Government White Paper, *The New NIIS, Modern, Dependable*, based on partnership and quality and driven by performance is music to the ears of many clinicians[14]. It is wonderful to hear the proposals for ICM with all care planners and providers working collaboratively and at last to have everyone singing from the same song sheet. Many healthcare professionals have been working with a number of health and social care organisations to develop programmes of care based on patient needs, expectations and outcomes. Multidisciplinary Pathways of Care© (MPC) is one of the risk management tools for monitoring the jointly agreed quality and patient outcome criteria. Integrated care is all about working in partnership, breaking down organisational, professional and territorial barriers by forging stronger links with health, social care, housing, education and employment bodies.

Table 2.2 Integrated care © 1996, Jo Wilson

☐ Incorporated multidisciplinary standards

☐ Processes linking to clinical outcomes

☐ Monitors and evaluates outcomes

☐ Patient and staff surveys

☐ Records variations/deviations from the care processes with real-time clinical audit

☐ Clinical guidelines are referred to or included

☐ The use of research, evidence-based practice and clinical effectiveness

Managed care

Managed care is a term that originated in the USA to describe a system of healthcare delivery that influences utilisation and cost of services, and measures performance. The goal is to have a plan that maximises value and is cost driven and financially controlled. The basic aim is to limit patients from over-consuming and providers from oversupplying. The managed care process in the UK and Europe is in its infancy and is causing some concerns in terms of driving down and containing costs and restrictions in clinical care. ICM is our chance in the UK to define clearly, document and communicate the care for our patients, and have clear criteria for monitoring based on good informed decision-making, patient needs and clinical outcomes. It provides a means by which the focus is quality driven, supported by purposeful clinical information which demonstrates efficiency and has ongoing measurements of performance.

ICM views the multidisciplinary approaches to collaborative care delivery by activity, cost and quality; and uses a process approach to problem- and outcome-based care delivery. It determines quality criteria by aligning clinical outcomes and financial responsibilities in the best interest of the patient and as part of the service level agreement between the planners and providers of care. Involving patients and their carers in determining the process and outcomes of care provides a route to better communication, patient and staff satisfaction, and the overall quality of care. ICM uses MPCs© as tools for minimising risk, changing practices and behaviours, and achieving continuous quality improvement of patient care. These objectives are achieved through better interdisciplinary working, coordinated care and promotion of patient-centred approaches. The result should be quick, reliable and appropriate service delivery.

Multidisciplinary pathways of care

Multidisciplinary pathways of care are defined as follows.

> MPCs© are multidisciplinary processes of patient focused care which specify key events, test and assessments, occurring in a timely fashion to produce the best prescribed outcomes, within the resources and activities available, for an appropriate episode of care[8].

MPCs© represent a process approach to managing integrated care to meet the individual needs of patients, and aligning clinical and financial responsibilities in their best interests. A pathway is a staged plan that notes the appropriate use of resources, the roles of professionals and the timing of procedures in relation to patient outcomes. The MPC© approach helps to reduce clinical variation in clinical practices across the different care settings, while continuing to maintain quality patient care and collaboration between care givers and to enhance clinical risk management. Currently there are at least 12 different nursing, medical and paramedical models of care each working to its own agenda

Vertical service delivery

Nursing	Medical	Paramedical

Screen ⇒ Assess ⇒ Plan ⇒ Implement ⇒

Patient fits into services ⇒ Evaluate against outcomes ⇒

Support services	Hotel services	Management services

All services impact on patient care but are often fragmented and uncoordinated

Figure 2.1   Vertical service delivery. © 1996, Jo Wilson.

producing a vertical system of care delivery (Figure 2.1), resulting in fragmented and uncoordinated processes, and the patient has to fit into the process. Integrated care works to a single multidisciplinary model of care (Figure 2.2) which moves with the patient across the different sectors of care; its usage is shared by different professional groups and between health and social care thereby reducing fragmentation in decision-making, and breaking down any boundaries or barriers to care delivery. The benefits achieved to date have been able to demonstrate that collaboration of seamless care reduces fragmentation and improves coordination and efficiency by reducing duplication, rework and wasting of resources (Figure 2.3). The MPC© model outlines the workforce requirements and makes clear the roles and responsibilities of professionals providing integrated care across all sectors including the patient's home.

A variance from the pathway is a deviation or detour from the multidisciplinary plan of care and these are to be expected due to individualised

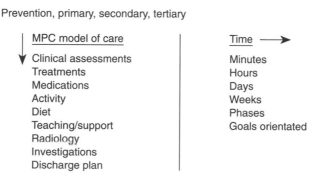

Pathway design - across the continuum of care

Prevention, primary, secondary, tertiary

MPC model of care	Time ⟶
Clinical assessments	Minutes
Treatments	Hours
Medications	Days
Activity	Weeks
Diet	Phases
Teaching/support	Goals orientated
Radiology	
Investigations	
Discharge plan	

Figure 2.2   Integrated care management. © 1996, Jo Wilson.

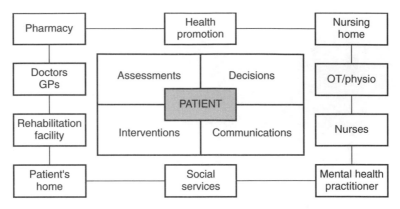

Figure 2.3   Integrated care management model. © 1996, Jo Wilson.

patient care explaining reasons for omissions and commissions in care. Variations from the pathway are immediately recorded and acted upon through the care management audit problem-solving process. These tools inquire into clinical practice and test out evidence-based care, quality criteria measurement and decision-making to identify remedial factors to improve practice. Variance analysis provides the 'window of opportunity' to indicate if things are missed/changed for specific patients and whether there are process or system failures thereby demonstrating individualised patient care and reasons for omissions and commissions. The MPC© is thus used as a means of determining and monitoring multidisciplinary standards of care, incorporating evidence-based practice and clinical effectiveness, patient/treatment outcomes and variations in care.

CLINICAL EFFECTIVENESS IMPROVEMENTS THROUGH EVIDENCE-BASED CARE AND PRACTICES

Improving clinical effectiveness clearly outlines the need for the multidisciplinary team to identify and develop evidence-based care and to develop and share best practices through clinical guidelines or protocols of care. The government plans for the setting up a new performance framework with an evidence-based national service framework, further research and development programmes, a commission for health improvement and an institute for clinical excellence will further enhance the work already undertaken and will promote uniformly high standards of excellence[15]. The opportunities these frameworks will provide will enhance integrated care by determining national clinical guidelines, variance codes and explicit quality standards which will provide excellent opportunities for clinical benchmarking between healthcare providers and sharing of best practices. An integrated care system focuses on the processes necessary for continuity of care, by examining the organisation and management of care, facilitating the smooth transition between hospital and home. Thus helps clinicians and managers to communicate the process thereby managing and reducing clinical risk and governance. Providing a risk management tool for clinical governance to ensure consistent standards, clinical indicators and performances are measured, clinical outcomes are evaluated and the processes identified in the MPC© are in place and monitored for continuous quality improvements.

MPCs© provide a framework giving greater quality assurance and proactive collaborative care through promoting timely, uniform quality and multidisciplinary standards, with a focus on continually learning from and improving the process. They incorporate patient and staff satisfaction surveys to demonstrate benefits realisation through better information, education, collaboration, documentation and communication of care delivery. They help trusts in their quest for continuous quality improvements by seeking better understanding and control of the care delivery process, achieving quality through efficient accountability and a better workforce through the promotion of recruitment and retention of staff.

HEALTHCARE RISK MANAGEMENT

Consistency in practice with reduced clinical variability is important for clinical, financial and organisational risk management. Managing the utilisation of healthcare resources in a systematic manner while maintaining or improving quality of clinical practice and patient outcomes effectively is necessary for integrated care efficiencies. The development and implementation of MPCs© designed by multidisciplinary teams can enable the integrated healthcare provider system to achieve this goal and meet the clinical governance requirements by ensuring standards are met and the processes are in place for continuous quality improvements. MPCs© improve communication and documentation of patient care. Currently care is recorded in various professional records up to eight times and communication is haphazard and inefficient; there is a need for an accurate and concise plan of care and a communication strategy. MPCs© provide this interdisciplinary record and communication tool promoting a collaborative care network which can start at diagnosis through any kind of health or social care setting and end back in the patient's home when the total episode of care is complete.

In the professional liability arena, standards of care issues span across the health and social care networks. Dual standards, when care is provided to the same patient to different standards, may produce threats of exposure to the networks overall. Many clinical negligence cases have used a dual standard of care within the same trust as an argument for plaintiff verdicts. Variances in the quality, standards of care and clinical practice within the health and social care organisations can create risk exposure leading to fragmented uncoordinated care and patient uncertainty. Practitioners have individual

Table 2.3 Healthcare risk management: clinical improvement model © 1996, Jo Wilson

Appropriateness	Efficiency	Effectiveness
Should it be done?	How to do it?	Did it work?
Clinical guidelines	Multidisciplinary Pathways of Care©	Clinical outcome measurement

responsibility and accountability for the quality of their practice as part of professional self-regulation.

The White Paper also addresses the question of appropriateness of care with the needs of patients being central to the system. Information to date has concentrated on quality alone, but as quality of care increases, the appropriateness of care decreases, resulting in unnecessary activities and inefficiency.

Integrated care through a healthcare improvement model (Table 2.3) can help to address these issues in the following ways.

- *Appropriateness of care* MPCs© define the practice parameters, addressing whether interventions should be done and how well they are done, compared to evidence-based medicine and clinical effectiveness. Outlining the health needs and requirements of individual patients is achieved by having MPCs© for different care groups and disease areas within the population. MPCs© also examine the process and sequence of care to ensure that they meet patient needs, interdisciplinary standards and outcome targets.
- *Efficiency* is determined by discussing and agreeing how and when to undertake the interventions to meet the quality criteria. *Does it pay its way?* Efficiency and quality go hand in hand to meet appropriateness of care ensuring best practices and utilisation of scarce resources.
- *Effectiveness* is determined from outcome measurement. *Did it work and is it worth doing?* Examination of effectiveness should compare outcome with patient and staff expectations. This will show whether care has been delivered appropriately, in a timely way and to the agreed quality criteria and interdisciplinary standards.

MPCs© decrease variability in outcomes, provide reproducible results and contribute to the development of quality assurance programmes providing benchmarks for clinical audit and sharing of best practices. They can assist the integrated care process by aiding the design of health improvement programmes which are able to demonstrate improvements in health and healthcare locally.

Integrated care and the use of the MPC© tool can also assist in the process of minimising or eliminating exposure to clinical risk through being a risk modification tool. Risk modification is the changing of circumstances, the environment and behaviour ultimately to lower the potential for healthcare risk. The result is improved outcomes, patient satisfaction and the documentation of patient care. They also comply with risk management which can be described as designing and directing activities that establish the conditions for organisation success within the context of service delivery.

Management must evaluate the effectiveness of clinical practice, patient satisfaction and outcomes and examine the frequency/defensibility of claims, MPCs© are one of the tools which can facilitate this system[8].

To improve continuously the clinical process quality, reduce risk and appropriately control efficiency it is essential to eliminate inappropriate variation and document continuous improvement. Improving integrated care based on partnership, quality, efficiency and performance is exactly the direction set out in the *New NHS* providing a modern and dependable service which is easily accessible and responsive.

CLINICAL RISK MODIFICATION

The tools of clinical risk modification are designed to be proactive and to concentrate on helping the multidisciplinary team to minimise and/or eliminate the causes of potential risks. They should be used to assist professionals in the audit and evaluation of their healthcare delivery with local ownership and control. They also serve as a change management mechanism for the healthcare organisation striving towards the best outcomes.

The main reasons why risks occur are highlighted in Table 2.4. Risks occur where the appropriate processes and systems are not clearly defined or short cuts are allowed or forced to take place due to workforce or organisational problems. Staff may not clearly be aware of their roles and responsibilities and be forced or pressurised to work beyond their skills and competency levels without the necessary education and training. The scope of professional practice has liberated the professions and allowed them to do much more to the benefits of patients. There must be a structured framework with a rationale,

---

Table 2.4 Why risks occur © 1994, Jo Wilson

- System failures
- Short cuts
- Communication breakdowns
- Ill-defined responsibilities
- Inadequately trained staff
- Inadequate policies, procedures, guidelines
- Poor interagency or interdepartmental working
- Dishonesty

education, training and development needs, skills and competency levels to be achieved and assessment and maintenance in terms of observation, supervised practice and competence; also the frequency and evaluation criteria to maintain the competency. No longer can we accept a 'see one, do one, teach one' approach, in the interest of professionalism, quality and risk management. They also identify communication and documentation issues including inter-agency and intradepartmental working. Dishonesty or cover-ups do also still exist due to fears of reporting, malingerers, people who do not learn lessons from mistakes and those who fortunately are few who wish to harm patients. Most of us do not deliberately go to work to harm or produce unwanted out-comes for patients/clients. Therefore when things to go wrong we need to identify the strengths and weakness, put things right and learn from the mistakes. The most important issue is to provide support for the patient and staff involved to help them cope and to help them through the process.

There are some key problem areas, according to claims and incident analysis. To achieve clinical risk modification we need to have risk identification and controls in these processes. Again they cover the communication and documen-tation areas and consent to treatment. (These will be covered in Chapters 6, 7, 8 and 9). Supervision of junior and trainee staff, including locums and new staff, is an important risk and quality issue in terms of the need for appropriate induction, orientation, education and ongoing training. Too often staff are left to undertake procedures where they do not have the skills, competency and supervision to do them safely. They may feel pressurised or afraid to ask or admit they have not done this before. One of the problem areas is when junior doctors are left unsupervised during middle and or senior grade study leave or holidays and no one is nominated to undertake the supervision. A clear chain of command policy is essential and a jump call policy for staff to contact the next more senior person to discuss decisions they are not happy with. This should be supported by a clear flow diagram outlining the policy and chain of command. (This will be discussed in further detail in Chapter 3).

It is essential that all grades of staff keep up-to-date with professional devel-opments, education and training to provide high-quality, low-risk care delivery (Table 2.5).

Table 2.5 Clinical risks: some key problem areas © 1994, Jo Wilson

- Communication and informed consent
- Supervision of junior staff
- Clinical record content and organisation
- Operating theatre procedures
- Timeliness of patient care
- Acting on pathology and imaging results
- Working beyond level of competence
- Locums and new staff

CONCLUSION

Clinical risk modification is the changing of circumstances, the environment and behaviour ultimately to lower the potential for and amount of healthcare risk. The result is improved outcomes, patient satisfaction and the documentation of care delivery. In the words of Ovretviet[16]:

> People and perfect processes make a quality health service – a poor quality service results from a badly designed and operated process, not from lazy or incompetent healthcare workers.

Yet how often in practice when things go wrong is there finger pointing and blame instead of support and guidance to staff? The process not the people make the system break down. A proactive risk modification process enables managers and the multidisciplinary team to control effectively the safety, activity, cost and quality of healthcare service delivery. There is an increasing move towards the need for better ICM with patient-centred care through improved communication and documentation. The best means of risk prevention is a comprehensive system for documenting, communicating and sharing patient care which is complete and related to the monitoring of standards and clinical outcomes through the real-time clinical audit process. An excellent way of achieving this standard, coordinating care and incorporating integrated care is through the use of clinical guidelines, evidence-based practice and MPCs©.

REFERENCES

1. Wilson, J. H. (1994) Quality in clinical care healthcare risk modification. *Health Business Summary*, **April.**
2. *The Pocket Oxford Dictionary* (1985) Oxford University Press: Oxford.
3. *The American College Dictionary* (1963) Random House: New York.
4. Williams, C. A. and Heins, R. M. (1976) *Risk Management and Insurance.* McGraw-Hill: New York.
5. Department of Health (1996) *Clinical Negligence Costs.* FDL (96)39. NHS Executive, DOH: Leeds.
6. Clinical Negligence Scheme for Trusts (1996) *Risk Management Standards and Procedures: Manual of Guidance.* CNST: Bristol.
7. Health Service Commissioner (1994) *Annual Report for 1993–4.* HMSO: London. Health Service Commissioner (1997) *Annual Report for 1997.* HMSO: London.
8. Wilson, J. H. (1992) *An Introduction to Multidisciplinary Pathways of Care.* Northern Regional Health Authority: Newcastle upon Tyne.
9. Audit Commission (1992) *Making time for Patients – A Handbook for Ward Sisters.* London. Audit Commission (1995) *Setting the Records Straight.* London. Audit Commission (1997) *Comparing Notes: A Study of Information Management in Community Trusts.* London.
10. Lester, G. W. and Smith, S. G. (1993) Listening and talking to patients. *West Journal of Medicine*, **158**, 268–272.

11. Engel, G. L. (1988) How much longer must medicine's science be bound by a seventeenth century world? In *The Task of Medicine: Dialog at Widkenburg* (K. L. While, ed.) Kaiser Family Foundation: USA.
12. Beckman, N. B. and Frankel, R. F. (1984) The effect of provider behaviour on the collection of data. *Annals of International Medicine,* **101**, 692–696.
13. Wilson, J. H. (1996) *Integrated Care Management: The Path to Success?* Butterworth-Heinemann: Oxford.
14. Department of Health (1997) *The New NHS, Modern, Dependable.* Cmnd 3807. HMSO: London.
15. NHS Executive (1998) *The New NHS Modern and Dependable: A National Framework for Assessing Performance.* 12394 FPA 5k 2P Feb 98 (RIC). HMSO: London.
16. Ovretviet, J. (1990) *Quality Health Service.* Brunel Institute of Organisational and Social Studies: London.

3 RISK REVIEWS AND USING RISK MANAGEMENT STRATEGY

Jo Wilson

INTRODUCTION

Healthcare delivery is a risky business. People are starting to view the NHS in the same light as other commercial businesses such as the hotel, retail and airline industries. The new White Paper *The New NHS, Modern, Dependable* places statutory responsibilities on managers and clinicians to provide a quality service and to be accountable for clinical governance and performance management[1]. The author firmly believes that quality and risk are two sides of the same coin, i.e. if you have good quality you have low risk, and this belief supports the clinical effectiveness agenda. Healthcare organisations in all sectors of care delivery need to demonstrate their high levels of achievement and commitment to continuous quality improvements. As discussed in Chapter 2, risk management is a process for the identification of risks that have adverse effects on the quality, safety and effectiveness of service delivery; the assessment and evaluation of those risks, and positive action to eliminate or reduce them. Effective clinical risk modification requires the application and monitoring of risk management standards; having a clear risk management strategy with an action plan; undertaking focused risk reviews in a systematic way across all specialties and departments; and having an effective incident reporting systems. This chapter will address in more detail each of these issues including the role of the Clinical Negligence Scheme for Trusts.

INTRODUCTION TO THE CLINICAL NEGLIGENCE SCHEME FOR TRUSTS

The Clinical Negligence Scheme for Trusts (CNST) is a mutual pooling pay-as-you-go arrangement for NHS Trusts in England[2]. It was designed to assist trusts in meeting the costs of clinical negligence claims, thereby optimising patient care and protecting the trust against the adverse consequences of clinical negligence. It is anticipated that over a period of years, depending on a number of factors including the claims experience, the trusts will meet the full costs of their clinical negligence liabilities. The CNST is administered by the National Health Service Litigation Authority (NHSLA) and is one of two schemes providing reimbursement to healthcare trusts in relation to clinical negligence claims. The other scheme, the Existing Liabilities Scheme (ELS), deals with cases arising from incidents before 1 April 1995 and is managed directly by the NHSLA and their solicitors. The intended impact of the CNST is to link risk management and claims management and to reduce the incidence of claims. Through promoting risk management standards (Table 3.1) it is hoped that best practice in risk and claims management will be established and that a national clinical negligence database will be built up. The CNST is now three years old; in terms of dealing with claims it is still early days, given the 'long scorpion tail' nature of clinical negligence claims which often take at least seven years to mature. The CNST has undoubtedly contributed to the improvements in risk management within the NHS with the setting up of risk management strategies and a series of focused risk reviews, particularly in the high-risk specialties.

A similar scheme has been set up in Wales and this is called 'The All Wales Risk Pool', which is currently answerable to the Welsh Office. The WRP covers both clinical and non-clinical claims. The excess is £30 000, although this is

Table 3.1 CNST risk management standards (reproduced from *CNST Risk Management Standards and Procedures Manual of Guidance*, April, 1996)

1. The board has a written risk management strategy that makes its commitment to managing clinical risk explicit.

2. An executive director of the board is charged with responsibility for clinical risk management throughout the trust.

3. The responsibility for management and coordination of clinical risk is clear.

4. A clinical incident reporting system is operated in all medical specialties and clinical support departments.

5. There is a policy for rapid follow up of major clinical incidents.

6. An agreed system of managing complaints is in place.

7. Appropriate information is provided to patients on the risks and benefits of the proposed treatment or investigation, and the alternatives available, before a signature on a consent form is sought.

8. A comprehensive system for the completion, use, storage and retrieval of medical records is in place. Record-keeping standards are monitored through the clinical audit process.

9. There is an induction/orientation programme for all new clinical staff.

10. A clinical risk management system is in place.

11. There is a clear documented system for management and communication throughout the key stages of maternity care.

Table 3.2   Welsh Risk Pool: risk management standards © WRP

Effective from 1 April 1999

There are 11 general standards

1. Risk profile
2. Risk management strategy
3. Incident reporting system
4. Patient records
5. Clinical audit
6. Complaints
7. Policies and procedures
8. Communications
9. Supervision of junior staff
10. Assessing competence
11. Health and safety, and related issues

There is one set of specialist standards for each of the following:

12A. Mental health
12B. Ambulance
12C. Operating theatres
12D. Accident and emergency
12E. Maternity
12F. Community

about to change to reflect the value of any individual case, and each hospital pays a premium into the fund which is related to the trust budget. The premiums are increasing sharply at present to cover liabilities carried by the WRP both of present trust claims and those of previous health authorities. The WRP is in the process of introducing risk management standards (Table 3.2) that are similar to, but by no means the same, as the CNST standards and which will be audited by the district audit function. The relative weightings for the 12 standards have been agreed by the WRP management group and are intended to reflect the relative importance of their effectiveness in reducing risk (Table 3.3). Financial incentives to award achievement of these standards are currently under development. The Welsh Office also, by means of a common services agency, provides legal support for trusts that wish to use these services. Arrangements in Scotland and Northern Ireland remain much as they were at the time of the introduction of Crown Indemnity. However, the inclusion of clinical risk management as a requirement for clinical governance in the White Paper would suggest that all parts of the UK will soon be taking part.

Table 3.3 Welsh Risk Pool: monitoring the risk management standards 1998/9 © WRP

The following relative weightings for the 12 standards have been agreed by the WRP Management

	Standards	Percentage
1.	Risk profile	14
2.	Risk management strategy	10
3.	Incident reporting	14
4.	Patient records	8
5.	Clinical audit	5
6.	Complaints	5
7.	Policies and procedures	8
8.	Communications	8
9.	Supervision of junior staff	8
10.	Assessing competence	10
11.	Health and Safety	10
Total		100

The weightings are intended to reflect the relative importance of the issue in terms of its effectiveness in risk.

THE SCHEMES

The schemes are aimed at promoting more effective risk, quality and claims management resulting in better standards of patient care. The emphasis is on the adoption of prudent risk management strategies; meeting the CNST and WRP risk management standards; implementing in full the new complaints procedure including its potential linkages to near misses, clinical indicators and clinical incidents to provide an alternative remedy for some potential litigants; and adopting a systematic approach to claims handling in line with best practice.

BACKGROUND TO THE CNST

The CNST was launched on 1 April 1995 and membership, currently over 400 trusts, of the scheme is voluntary and its primary purpose is to give greater certainty to budgeting and planning by providing financial assistance to trusts in the event of a very large claim, a run of high claims or a serial claim, any of which could otherwise cause severe financial problems. The CNST and WRP were created specifically to protect trusts against the effects of the higher and relatively infrequent clinical negligence claims. Trusts can choose to have one of six excess levels depending on their specialties, income, claims management and history. A discount of 5 per cent in this first year was awarded on the basis of a completed self-assessment questionnaire and evidence of progress in implementing clinical risk management standards from supporting documentation.

ESSENTIAL PRINCIPLES OF THE CNST

Risk management standards (see Table 3.1) were launched in April 1996; they will form the basis of an annual assessment visit which will determine future discounts. The standards are aimed at ensuring that risk management is conducted in a focused and effective fashion which is intended to have a positive contribution towards the improvement of patient care within member trusts. Eleven basic CNST standards have been developed, 10 of which are core standards and number 11 refers to maternity care. Compliance with these standards will be monitored and scored on three levels, reflecting as closely as possible the relative difficulty in attaining the level and each level having to be achieved before being assessed at the next level. Only one assessment of a member can be made in any one scheme year. The level one standards were basic risk management procedures which enabled the CNST member to obtain an initial 5 per cent discount on contributions. These standards included a written and formally agreed risk management strategy from the trust board, a full or part-time risk manager in post, and a clinical risk management system and incident reporting system in place. Level two and level three standards (Table 3.4) are more difficult and will take longer to achieve and must be supported by 90 per cent continued compliance with level one standards.

Each standard has a number of key features which are scored and weighted according to relevant importance to risk management and the different levels of achievement. While the standards are not intended to be comprehensive, they are designed in such a way that every trust can use them to develop its own comprehensive risk management strategy and risk reviews.

Claims assessment standards, procedures and guidelines have been drawn up by the CNST to ensure that payments made are justified, appropriate and equitable to all members in terms of good claims handling and management within individual trusts. The NHS Litigation Authority framework document draws upon the standards, procedures and guidelines with the aim of ensuring that genuine claimants receive an appropriate remedy[3]. Currently there is considerable variability in the way quantum and costs are estimated, but over time it is expected that discrepancies will be ironed out as claims handlers become more familiar with the process. In the summer of 1997 there were 634 open claims with an estimated settlement value of £180m, with the incidents incurred but not reported (INBR) the total could increase to £500m, with an overall liability (pre–post trust) estimated at £1 to £3 billion. It is a declared aim of the NHSLA to speed up the litigation process and to encourage dialogue between the defence and plaintiff solicitors. The more open each party is able to be the sooner each party will be able to make a proper assessment of its case and the sooner the case will be resolved. The NHSLA also suggest

Table 3.4 CNST risk management standards: three levels (reproduced from *CNST Risk Management Standards and Procedures Manual of Guidance*, April, 1996)

Standard	No. of criteria	Level of standard to be met
1. The board has a written risk management strategy that makes its commitment to managing clinical risk explicit.	6	1, 2 and 3
2. An executive director of the board is charged with responsibility for clinical risk management throughout the trust.	2	Both level 1
3. The responsibility for management and coordination of clinical risk is clear.	2	Both level 1
4. A clinical incident reporting system is operated in all medical specialities and clinical support departments.	16	8 at level 1 6 at level 2 2 at level 3
5. There is a policy for rapid follow up of major clinical incidents.	8	6 at level 1 1 at level 2 1 at level 3
6. An agreed system of managing complaints is in place.	3	1, 2, and 3
7. Appropriate information is provided to patients on the risks and benefits of the proposed treatment or investigation, and the alternatives available, before a signature on a consent form is sought.	5	2 at level 1 2 at level 2 1 at level 3
8. A comprehensive system for the completion, use, storage and retrieval of medical records is in place. Record-keeping standards are monitored through the clinical audit process.	18	9 at level 1 6 at level 2 3 at level 3
9. There is an induction/orientation programme for all new clinical staff.	8	3 at level 1 3 at level 2 2 at level 3
10. A clinical risk management system is in place.	5	4 at level 2 1 at level 3
11. There is a clear documented system for management and communication throughout the key stages of maternity care.	10	5 at level 1 2 at level 2 3 at level 3

that a regular internal audit should be carried out by the trust to ensure that they meet the specified minimum standards within their claims handling procedures. In February 1998 the health secretary Frank Dobson pledged to the Lord Chancellor to keep lawyers out of hospital, and doctors out of court. In March 1998 the Lord Chancellor proposed arrangements to manage negligence claims better in a Green Paper which put a figure at £27m spent on legal aid in funding plaintiff cases against the NHS. In May 1998 Frank Dobson was quoted as saying[4]:

We've got to raise standards in the NHS. We've also got to make the NHS more helpful and responsive to patients when things go wrong so fewer people will feel the need to turn to the lawyers. We want explanation, not litigation. Apologies, not accusations. Excellence, not excuses.

According to Sanderson each year the CNST collects enough money to pay the actual damages and costs which fall due to be paid in that year[5]. Contributions are based on actuarial advice and reflect the type of NHS trust involved and its range of services. In due course when a claims history becomes meaningful, this will be the basis on which the subscription is calculated. A basis principle of the CNST is that members should always contribute to each claim settlement and the scheme has been designed in such a way that trusts pay 100 per cent of the value of claims up to a chosen excess. For claims above the chosen excess up to a linked ultimate threshold the trust makes a contribution of 20 per cent. Above the ultimate threshold the scheme will pay the balance of any claim.

As from the 1 April 1998, the claims management system will change for all new cases relating to the CNST (there is no change regarding the ELS, or cases involving the CNST pre-1 April 1998). Under the new system, trusts and health authorities will no longer appoint their own solicitors in clinical negligence cases relating to the CNST, but instead the NHSLA will instruct solicitors on their behalf. There will be a panel of 18 defendant solicitor firms initially and the NHSLA will set standards, protocols and fees and will manage the litigation centrally. The will help the NHSLA to fulfil its three aims which are: to settle justified claims for a reasonable sum as soon as practicable; to defend unjust claims robustly; and to make a judgement about which course to choose in an individual case by considering the likely outcome in court. Steve Walker, the Chief Executive of the NHSLA, is quoted as saying[4]:

Our experience is that claims are not handled well, for a number of reasons. More than 90 firms of solicitors are listed as doing medical defence work for the NHS, and the quality of their work ranges from the professionally negligent to perfectly satisfactory – and I'm not saying brilliant. The NHSLA is now instituting proceedings against one firm.

CNST RISK MANAGEMENT STANDARDS

As outlined in Table 3.1, the standards are focused upon the organisational, communication and documentation issues, which are all related to the prevention and minimisation of risk exposure. A clear chain of command with individual roles and responsibilities ensures that the risks are managed and reflected in the commitment of the trust board members. This ensures that policies, procedures and clinical guidelines are updated to maintain safe systems of work for patients, staff and visitors. Staff are orientated and inducted appropriately to the organisation at trust and specialty levels and this also refers

Table 3.5 Contingent liability by speciality © 1997 CNST

Speciality	Value £ million
Accident and emergency	2.3
Anaesthetics	2.9
General surgery	2.1
Gynaecology	1.2
General medicine	1.6
Paediatrics	2.9
Obstetrics	59.1
Orthopaedics	1.6
Cardiac surgery	1.5
Others	6.0
Total	81.2

to locums, bank and agency staff. Informed consent receives a high weighting at all levels with an increased need for providing information leaflets and communicating with patients the risks, alternatives and benefits of all invasive procedures.

There is an increasing move towards the need for better integrated care management (ICM) (as discussed in Chapter 2) with patient-centred care through improved communication and documentation[6]. This is the best means of risk prevention. ICM provides a comprehensive system for documenting, communicating and sharing patient care which is related to the monitoring of standards and clinical outcomes through the real-time clinical audit process. An excellent way of achieving this standard, coordinating care and incorporating interdisciplinary care is through the use of clinical guidelines and Multi-disciplinary Pathways of Care© (MPCs©)[7]. This methodology and its benefits as a risk management tool are included in Chapter 2.

The CNST/WRP are voluntary schemes enabling trusts and health authorities to pool the cost of clinical negligence settlements each year in return for an annual subscription. Bearing in mind that prevention is cheaper than cure, the potential risk/clinical negligence exposure by specialty is outlined in Table 3.5 which provides the contingent liability from the CNST.

In time the CNST should have a powerful database on risk and claims management and be able to identify significant trends in litigation. This will provide powerful information which can be used proactively in terms of clinical effectiveness, benchmarking by clinical indicators, the production of appropriate guidelines incorporated in MPCs© and informing education and training programmes.

RISK REVIEWS TO ACHIEVE RISK MODIFICATION

There are two main types of risk review: one is a comprehensive risk review and the other is a focused risk review. The reasons why risks occur need to be considered in all types of reviews. The generic reasons why risks occur (as discussed briefly in Chapter 2) include the following:

- System failures with lack of clearly defined processes, policies, procedures and clinical guidelines resulting in errors or slips and lapses of memory.
- Staff taking short cuts for a number of reasons including heavy and uncontrolled workload, pressures of work and suffering from stress through feeling lack of support. These can lead to mistakes where the wrong actions can be undertaken, violations including deliberate acts or active failures resulting in unsafe acts by individuals.
- Communication breakdowns between the healthcare practitioners, with outside agencies and with patients and relatives resulting in poor quality of care delivery.
- Ill-defined responsibilities where staff are unsure whose role it is and who has the skills and competencies to undertake certain procedures and activities. Often staff can feel pressurised to increase their scope of professional practice without the necessary education, skills training and proficiencies/competencies to undertake the responsibilities.
- Inadequately trained staff who are not given ongoing education and training to keep up-to-date, maintain their skills and competency levels, develop clinical guidelines and evidence-based practice, to undertake critical appraisals and to establish and maintain clinical effectiveness.
- Inadequate policies and procedures which do not provide enough information and guidance for staff and cause latent failures which provides an environment which is conducive to failures occurring.
- Poor interagency or interdepartmental working where information is not shared and there is no appreciation of each others agendas or pressures of work resulting in fragmentation and uncoordinated care delivery
- Dishonesty which results in practitioners deliberately wanting to interrupt the system or damage the patients.

Reviews can highlight the possible areas where things might go wrong and devise processes and systems to be put in place to minimise or eliminate the potential risks. Having adequate reporting systems can identify near misses, complaints, incidents and potential/actual claims for lessons to be learned, and practice, behaviour and cultural changes to be made.

COMPREHENSIVE RISK REVIEW AND A RISK MANAGEMENT STRATEGY REPORT FOR THE ORGANISATION

The comprehensive review is a top level review involving the senior managers and clinicians within the organisation. The idea is to identify organisation-wide problems for strategic change and ongoing review. It can also identify specific areas within specialties which need to be subject to a more focused risk review of that particular clinical unit. The process varies depending on the type and level of care delivery of the organisation, in terms of the people who are requested for interview, the documents reviewed, the areas selected for inspection and the types of checklists used with different priorities and emphasis.

Methodology used

The basis of the comprehensive risk review is a process which ensures that evidence of potential risk exposures is corroborated through the following methodology. First a walkabout/tour of the trust/healthcare facilities is undertaken. Second, an audit tool is used with the documentation provided to identify additional areas of concern and areas at which to target the interview questions. This includes a review of randomly selected, organisation-wide, patient records which are audited using a comprehensive checklist. Third, interviews are undertaken with the top-level managers and clinicians within the organisation. The results are summarised into areas of concern which are mentioned by more than one individual or through verification within the documentation review. Once all areas of potential risk exposure are identified there is the need to develop a series of high level recommendations to address each risk exposure. These recommendations are then grouped into a manageable number of categories in three groups: administration, services/systems and workforce issues. A draft report is then produced for initial discussion with the risk management committee. After this discussion, revisions are made to the report and it is submitted to the hospital management committee.

A final report will then be issued and presented to the interviewees. Action planning will be undertaken with these people to allow local ownership and control of the recommendations, with review and evaluation dates. This document should be viewed as a confidential communication for the purpose of improving the delivery of patient care. The hospital may wish to share this report with appropriate individuals who have a need to know and use it as a mechanism to stimulate discussion at risk management and clinical audit meetings. It may also be used for education purposes. In each instance, this clinical risk management strategy is intended to help the individual hospital to minimise potential risk exposures, and actively manage those adverse events that do occur.

FOCUSED RISK REVIEW RESULTING IN A STRATEGY REPORT FOR A PARTICULAR SPECIALITY, DEPARTMENT OR CLINICAL UNIT

The focused risk review is a specialty-specific review. Examples of those undertaken on a regular basis are: accident and emergency services; obstetrics and gynaecology; operating theatres; anaesthetics and ICUs; neurosciences; surgical services; orthopaedic and trauma services; community services; mental health; occupational health; control of infection; medical unit services including bed management; paediatric services; health and safety compliance and audits; patients' medical records review including storage, retrieval and retention; renal services; and the integration of health and social care. These involve all grades and levels of management, clinical and support staff within the specialty. The idea is to identify specialty-specific problems with the adequacy, compliance, awareness and knowledge of processes and systems set up for patients', staff and visitors' safety and the minimisation of risks. This results in a report again based on high level recommendations, detailed issues raised and discussion for implementation, action planning and ongoing review and evaluation.

Methodology used

The basis for the recommendations is a process which ensures that evidence of potential risk exposures is corroborated through the following methodology. First there is a comprehensive specialty-specific documentation review including policies, procedures, guidelines and MPCs©; open and closed clinical negligence and employee liability claims analysis; the 3Cs (complaints, compliments and comments) quarterly reports; incidents over the past year; summed data on adherence to clinical indicators; and patients' medical records review of 10 cases selected by high-risk selection criteria and 30 cases selected at random from patients treated in the last six months. Second, a walkabout/tour of the specialty and all of its support services is undertaken. Third, a series of interviews are undertaken and are summarised and the areas of concern which are mentioned by more than one individual or verified in the documents or tour are noted. Fourth, time is spent in the unit/specialty tracking patient movement and observing practices. Analysis of the information received and application of a risk management index are used to prioritise the risk issues and the recommendations.

Once all areas of potential risk are identified there is a need to develop a series of recommendations to address the risk exposure. These recommendations are then grouped into a manageable number of categories in three areas: management, services/systems and workforce issues. A draft report is then produced for initial discussion with persons identified by the hospital/ NHS trust. This is verified and action planning is undertaken. This ensures that the specialty staff own, control and feel responsible for the implementation of the recommendations and areas to minimise risk exposure.

In all risk reviews it is important not to try to dissuade clinicians from taking risks, but to try to change individual behaviour when, inevitably, risks occur. This is very hard to do as it often needs cultural, individual and management changes to alter practice to reduce risk and modify behaviour. This can be obtained through risk awareness, risk identification, review of practices, changes in practices and ongoing evaluation. The benefits which the NHS trusts receive are in the format of an objective review which has been obtained by experts helping in the risk awareness, identification, audit criteria and ongoing evaluation. Often the issues raised can be consistent with some of the senior staff's feelings of deficiencies within the trust but to have them formalised within a document can help to put pressure on the organisation to change. The whole process of the awareness and evaluation; education and implementation and integration and support is all about developing ownership, control and actions around the issues as demonstrated below. Teaching staff to analyse their concerns and potential problems in this kind of way supports the minimisation of risk, modification of practitioner's behaviour and the integration of quality and clinical audit into daily practice.

RISK MANAGEMENT STRATEGY

A risk management strategy provides the framework for the development of a rigorous risk management process throughout the healthcare organisation. It acknowledges that whilst by its very nature healthcare is a risk activity, it is of considerable concern that a wide range of risks can occur by accident, mishap and mistake. Even more worrying are those untoward incidents which result from such deficiencies as the lack of clear policies of care, deficient working practices, poorly defined responsibilities, inadequate communications and other systems failures. The challenge for the managers, clinicians and all other staff within the trust is to eliminate, or at least reduce, the potential for such misfortunes by being more positive in the future management of risk.

The implementation of the risk management strategy should not be seen as simply another initiative demanding scarce managerial and clinical time. Instead, it should be regarded as part of the existing continuous quality improvement, business planning and organisational development agendas, embracing the following specific organisation initiatives.

- Identify opportunities to improve patient care.
- Identify opportunities to improve patient satisfaction.
- Improve the quality of care of patients and staff.
- Produce better integrated care with demonstrable clinical effectiveness.
- Identify opportunities to improve care communication and joint working.
- Identify opportunities to reduce the potential for untoward incidence occurrence.
- Health and safety action plan.

Risk management concerns the identification and analysis of risks, and the planning and implementation of control measures (physical, clinical, financial, cultural) to eliminate, reduce or transfer risk. Whilst the term 'hazard' denotes the potential to cause harm, 'risk' reflects the likelihood that harm will occur (i.e., probability, severity and frequency). Risk is the potential for an unwanted or unexpected outcome. A risk is anything which will harm the well-being and/ or assets of an individual or an organisation. Those risks which cannot be avoided must be reduced to an acceptable level. The costs associated with risks can be high, both in direct and indirect terms. It has been estimated that indirect costs can account for four times those of direct financial losses. Risk control concerns the prevention and correction of unsafe conditions and circumstances in respect of both individuals and the local environment. This requires planned, immediate and long term approaches. Risk prevention has been defined by Helmrech as[9]:

> . . . an integrated programme, a series of coordinated activities directed to the control of unsafe personal performance and unsafe mechanical conditions and based on certain knowledge, attitudes and abilities.

The constituent parts of successful risk management in the healthcare organisation are:

- a rigorous organisational framework to coordinate and oversee risk management activities;
- a learning organisational culture;
- managers, clinicians and staff who, through appropriate training and education, are constantly aware of their risk management responsibilities;
- interdisciplinary working through ICM and seamless care which follows the patient across the different sectors of care and into their home environment;
- an effective communication strategy supported by good documentation of policies, procedures, MPCs© and clinical guidelines which are reflected in the documentation of care given to patients; and
- the collection and analysis of information and the subsequent review and development of more risk-free operational practices and systems. Information sources include: risk assessments, audit data, clinical and non-clinical incident reporting and user feedback.

Risk management must be seen as an essential component of the organisation's continuous quality improvement programmes embracing good working practices, processes and systems. A key to successful risk management is to embed within the organisation the routine collection of information, its analysis and the subsequent feedback and appropriate action by clinicians and managers. Most organisations are starting to show great awareness of the risks facing it, both from internal and external sources, particularly in respect of business, contracting and health and safety issues, with emphasis increasingly being placed on the identification of clinical risk and its management. The organisation's board must be supportive of, and committed to, the further development of a risk management culture.

Commendably, many organisations have given named responsibility for risk management to a board executive director and some have appointed a risk manager with a clinical background to coordinate the activities with the emphasis on risk management being part of every staff member's role and responsibility. Consideration should also be given to linking the clinical risk, audit and quality processes to ensure maximisation of clinical risk modification. Through integrating these processes and having the right working group structures to report to the risk management steering group the organisation can demonstrate a framework for communication and coordination of the risk activities. This includes the use of clear simple definitions for near misses, incidents, critical incidents and clinical indictors and the use of a single easy to complete document which reports the same.

The organisation must then determine how it needs to demonstrate to users, staff and purchasers that, through the development and implementation of an organisation-wide risk management strategy, all reasonable steps are being taken, and will continue to be taken, to eliminate, reduce or transfer identified risks. The organisation should recognise that effective risk management is essential to the well-being of individual patients, residents and staff, as well as to the corporate governance of the organisation. Consequently, it is keen to develop positive risk management at all levels and within all services in the organisation, achieved through:

- increased staff awareness of all aspects of risk management;
- clarification of risk management roles and responsibilities;
- a desire to link audit, quality, clinical effectiveness and risk management activities to demonstrate continuous improvements in patient care;
- allocation of resources; and
- the development and auditing of risk management standards.

At the heart of these fundamental purposes and goals is the organisation's board's desire to create services which have their risks minimised, are secure for patients and clients and which provide a healthy and safe environment for the organisation's staff. The board is also aware of its legal and statutory obligations. NHS trusts are legally required to accept vicarious liability for the actions of all their staff and are held accountable for defending alleged cases of clinical negligence. Similarly, the trust and its officers are subject to potential criminal prosecution for breaches of legislative duties established to protect employees and the public from actions carried out in the normal course of the trust's activities. Accordingly, the trust board believes that by approaching the control of such risks in a strategic and organised manner, the risks can be reduced to an acceptable level. A key part of the strategy is a clear communication and documentation process and systems for review, monitoring and evaluation of their effectiveness. This will result in better quality care for patients and residents, a safer environment and a reduction in unnecessary expenditure. The use of a risk management strategy document should be designed for all managers and clinicians within the organisation to make it clear what are their responsibilities and opportunities for risk reduction and control.

The multidisciplinary team can begin to apply risk management to its own healthcare setting and achieve risk modification through the following.

- *Awareness and evaluation.* An in-depth assessment of the organisation's services and practices, and costs related to each, can begin to provide data from which potential risk areas can be identified. Included in this identification process are both the clinical and non-clinical components of the organisation that contribute to the overall episode of care. Awareness is the first phase of risk modification.
- *Education and implementation.* Development of processes and interventions that begin to change the undesirable practices of systems identified is the second phase of risk modification. This combines specific structural and procedural changes to be implemented, with an educational process for all involved.

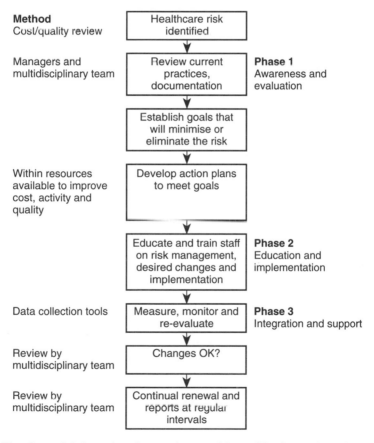

Figure 3.1 The flow of information for continuous risk modification and total quality improvements in the system of healthcare delivery.

● *Integration and support*. Once changes and interventions are decided upon, a system for monitoring their integration into the organisation is needed to determine if the change has actually reduced – modified – the identified risk. The data collection, analysis, measurement, monitoring and re-evaluation is the third part of risk modification.

This can be shown as a flow of activity (Figure 3.1) that fosters continuous risk modification and total quality improvements in the system of healthcare delivery.

To approach the process of healthcare risk management systematically, it is helpful to think in terms of the following four-step model for risk management:

1. The identification of risk.
2. The analysis of the risks identified.
3. The treatment of risk.
4. The evaluation of risk treatment strategies.

Risk identification

Risk identification is the process through which the healthcare organisation becomes aware of the risks in the healthcare environment that constitute potential loss exposures for the healthcare organisation. Identification and assessment of risk is an ongoing process with the objective of improved prevention, control and containment of risks. The risk management committees can use many information sources to identify potential risks. *Incident reporting is the cornerstone of most risk management systems.* Effective management of incidents will be achieved through the early identification of incidents, mistakes and 'near misses' and promptly and positively managing the effects of these.

Risk analysis

Risk analysis is the process of determining the potential severity of the loss associated with an identified risk and the probability that such a loss will occur. A defined system of effective complaints and claims management is essential and this will be achieved through the expeditious management of complaints and claims, thus reducing the costs, stress to staff and the patient/public hostility. These factors taken together establish the seriousness of a risk and guide the healthcare organisation's selection of an appropriate risk management strategy.

Risk treatment

Risk treatment refers to the range of choices available to the healthcare organisation in handling a given risk. Risk strategies include the following:

- risk control;
- risk acceptance;
- risk avoidance;
- risk reduction or minimisation; and
- risk transfer.

In addition to exploring these risk treatment strategies individually, the health-care organisation can fashion the combination of strategies that is best suited to managing a given risk exposure.

Risk control

It is acknowledged that it will not always be possible to eliminate risks entirely. Therefore, control measures will be instigated to reduce the likelihood of an adverse occurrence or outcome.

Primary risk reduction control will be achieved through one or more of the following measures:

- the development of a comprehensive risk assessment process;
- the development of a risk management training and education programme;
- the utilisation of policies, procedures, protocols, pathways and clinical guidelines, which if regularly reviewed, updated, formally introduced and complied with will provide guidance to help staff produce required out-comes which are consistent and reliable. Copies of outdated or superseded policies will be filed centrally and retained since they may be essential for the defence of a practice undertaken in the past; and
- contingency and disaster planning, which is important for reducing the affects of major internal incidents (e.g. loss of utilities).

Risk acceptance

One strategy for managing an identified risk is risk acceptance. Risk acceptance involves assuming the potential losses associated with a given risk and making plans to cover any financial consequences of such losses.

Risk acceptance is most appropriate for managing:

- those risks that cannot be otherwise reduced, transferred, or avoided; and
- those for which the probability of loss is great and the potential con-sequences are not beyond the healthcare organisation's ability to self-fund.

Risk avoidance

Risk avoidance through utilising alternatives represents another risk treatment strategy. When a given risk poses a particularly serious threat that cannot be effectively reduced or transferred, the conduct or service giving rise to the risk may perhaps be avoided.

Table 3.6 A sample action plan for risk modification

ACTION PLAN

CLINICAL RISK MODIFICATION STRATEGY PLAN: RECOMMENDATION NO. 1

IDENTIFIED RECOMMENDATION TOPIC	S–T M–T L–T	SUGGESTED ACTIONS TO BE ADDRESSED	LEAD MEMBER OF STAFF RESPONSIBLE AND OTHERS TO ASSIST	REVIEW DATES, TIME FRAME AND RESOURCES REQUIRED 1998/99

© Jo Wilson 1992[7]

Risk reduction or minimisation
Risk reduction or minimisation involves various loss control strategies aimed at limiting the potential consequences or frequency of a given risk without totally accepting or avoiding the risk. Risk reduction or minimisation efforts are at the heart of most healthcare organisation risk management programmes and include such activities as staff education, policy and procedure revision, and other interventions aimed at controlling adverse occurrences without completely eschewing potential risky activities.

Risk transfer
Risk transfer techniques involve shifting the risk of loss to another entity, either through the contracting process or by setting up a pooling arrangement with other healthcare organisations, e.g. the CNST and WRP. Financial savings will be achieved through increased proficiency in the utilisation of available resources, a reduction in the amount of duplicated effort and lower insurance premiums. Through continuing to undertake risk management activity the healthcare organisation may be able to demonstrate reductions in risk which can lead to reduction in premiums and loss exposure.

The healthcare organisation should employ a combination of risk treatment strategies, for most identified risks, to best manage a given situation. Contingency and disaster planning are also important in the reduction of the affects of major internal incidents and potential loss of utilities.

Risk management evaluation

The final step in the risk management process is risk management evaluation, whereby the effectiveness of the techniques employed to identify, analyse, and treat risks is gauged and assessed. Risk evaluation involves the risk management committee, the chief executive and healthcare organisation board members, the medical staff, all clinicians and legal/patient ombudsman/advocate. The multidisciplinary approach to evaluating the effectiveness of risk management programme ensures that the impact of the various risk management activities is measured accurately and that additional risk management activities are fully explored. Effective risk management is best achieved through an environment of honesty and openness, where mistakes and untoward events are identified quickly and dealt with in a positive and responsive way. A blame-free culture for reporting and dealing with events is advisable.

To facilitate the risk management evaluation process, the healthcare organisation needs to prepare a comprehensive annual report of risk management activities and an evaluation of the ongoing review of the action plan. The risk management strategy is personalised and updated through the evaluation process and the action planning is an essential ingredient; a sample plan is included in Table 3.6.

INCIDENT REPORTING

Having an open, honest and blame-free organisation which is open to improving processes and systems of care is a big step towards having staff committed to quality and getting things right. Near-miss, incident and indicator recording and reporting are the cornerstone of any quality and risk management system.

Incident reporting, investigation and follow up are considered a minimum, level one standard of the Clinical Negligence Scheme for Trusts, alongside the clinical complaints procedure providing a means of assessing areas where improvements need to be made. The reporting of near misses is also important as we can learn from these and put systems in place to stop them happening. A definition of a near miss may be 'an occurrence which but for luck or skilful management would in all probability have become an incident'. As healthcare professionals we need to be prepared to share things that have the potential to go wrong and to have a learning culture to prevent patient accident or injuries from occurring in the first place.

A clinical incident may be defined as 'any occurrence which is not consistent with the professional standards of care of the patient or the routine operation/ policies of the organisation'[10]. The CNST describes an incident as 'an unexpected event occurring during treatment, or unexpected result of treatment, which may, or does, cause harm to the patient'[11]. Experience to date has shown that a 1000-bed NHS trust with a bed occupancy of 89 per cent can expect to have 5800 clinical incidents per year, of which 116 have the potential for some form of compensation, and around 38 of these could become clinical negligence claims[10]. None of us, apart from a few malign individuals who invade the organisations, get out of bed in the morning and deliberately set out to harm or injure any patient. Yet we all know that in dealing with people it is inevitable that some accidents/incidents do occur.

Some of the pitfalls and failings of the common incident reporting systems are:

- due to some activities being given low priority, the failure of staff to identify serious events;
- the fear of reporting perceptions with finger pointing and blame being applied instead of support and help to put things right;
- punitive response especially for some disciplines such as nursing where many incidents result in disciplinary action; and
- having the wrong systems or inadequate policies, procedures and guidelines in the first place.

Each trust should have a clear definition of clinical incidents and should encourage reporting with an open and honest culture without the threat of punitive responses, and speciality-specific as well as trust-wide examples of what constitutes a near miss and incident should serve as a guide. Many trusts have undertaken this with the support of a letter to every member of staff from the chief executive reinforcing a 'blame-free culture' and highlighting that no member of staff will be disciplined unless an incident is malicious, criminal, keeps reoccurring without lessons being learned or constitutes gross professional misconduct. It is extremely important that near misses and incidents are tracked and trended to allow information to support the lessons which need to be learned, inform the education and training programmes and revise policies, procedures and guidelines building on the strengths of where things go right and analysing and improving the areas of weaknesses. Recording of incident information within a database and investigating events in a timely manner allows appropriate action to be set within a clear time frame to limit damages and prevent recurrences through reviewing practices and procedures and providing feedback to staff.

The places where incidents occur were broken down across one district as follows[12].

- Theatre: 32 per cent.
- Ward: 26 per cent.
- Accident and emergency department: 22 per cent.
- Outpatients: 18 per cent.
- Other: 2 per cent.

The areas very much focus around places where patients pass through the healthcare system and are reliant on good communication and documentation. The perioperative period is a particularly difficult area in these respects, due to the fact the patient is sedated or anaesthetised and has to rely on staff being the advocate for the patient with adequate checks to ensure that the right patient is in the right place at the right time and having the correct procedure.

CLINICAL INDICATORS

Clinical indicators (see also Chapters 2 and 4) which are specialty-specific early warning signs of things which need further review or investigation are an important component of clinical incident recording. These clinical indicators are based on the analysis of clinical negligence claims which identify common activities where things do go wrong. Clinical indicators provide:

- 'top of the trees' triggers or early warning signs which look at events that serve as a flag for deeper review through the clinical audit and effectiveness processes;
- timely comparative data sources with potential bench marking opportunities with other specialties in other trusts on a national basis to allow sharing and implementation of best practices and lessons learned; and
- support for decision making and promotion of behaviour change as necessary which is one of the most important components of risk management. If behaviour and practices do not change then accidents and litigation will continue to be a drain on the healthcare resources.

Examples of some organisation-wide clinical indicators are the following:

- an unexpected or trauma-related death;
- a neurological deficit not present on admission;
- coma not present on admission;
- disfigurement present on discharge, which was not present on admission, including amputation;
- unplanned returns to the operating theatre;
- unplanned admission to or the need for intensive care;
- failure to act upon imaging or pathology results;
- imaging or pathology reports to the wrong patient;
- adverse prescribing, administration and side effects of medications;
- equipment failure leading to patient injury or death;
- swab/needle/instrument count incorrect at the end of a procedure; and
- absent patient records.

Source: HRRI 1996

Effective near miss, clinical incident and indicator systems can provide essential information for education and development of staff; improvements in trust documentation for improving clinical practice; early identification of potential risk of clinical negligence cases, including the provision of details including statements from staff involved and location of their whereabouts; and an estimation of defensibility, liability and early settlement of potential or actual claims against the trust. Incident reporting, complaints and claims management need to be brought together under one umbrella to allow effective information to inform the risk management processes and to allow them to become much more proactive than reactive supporting the notion that prevention is cheaper than cure and certainly better for the patient in terms of quality of care.

HIGH-RISK SPECIALTIES

As demonstrated in the contingent liability table from the CNST, some specialties are more risky than others according to their claims profile. This table highlights obstetrics as being the most high-risk specialty with the others being fairly closely correlated. The current difficulties are that within the UK we do not have a good database to learn from claims to establish good clinical risk modification programmes. This is due to lack of central coordination and sharing of data. This should improve over time as the CNST database builds up and becomes more meaningful. Meanwhile the author undertook a review of closed claims which were available through firms of solicitors, law journals, the General Medical Council and some hospitals. These claims came from across the UK between March 1993 and July 1995 and numbered 401 closed claims. The analysis by specialty revealed the following:

- obstetrics, 101 cases, 25 per cent;
- gynaecology, 57 cases, 14.2 per cent;
- orthopaedics, 49 cases, 12.2 per cent;
- anaesthetics, 43 cases, 10.7 per cent;
- accident and emergency, 30 cases, 7.5 per cent;
- general surgery, 28 cases, 7.0 per cent.

The Scottish Office published data on 1185 cases which were open in August 1995, which revealed a similar pattern.

- obstetrics and gynaecology, 27 per cent;
- accident and emergency, 17 per cent;
- orthopaedics, 13 per cent;
- general surgery, 12 per cent.

The cost of litigation is continuing to rise in the UK. For the 401 closed claims the total of damages awarded was £23 909 596, a median of £59 182 per case, plus legal costs in all cases. Of the total costs of the awards, 38 per cent was for obstetric claims £6 876 033 and for gynaecology the amount was £2 413 124. The average cost for an obstetric claim was £68 080 and it was £42 335 for gynaecology, clearly demonstrating that these are the most high-risk specialties.

A further analysis of the claims by specialty brought up a number of factors specific to each.

Obstetrics

In obstetrics the following features were noted.

- A high proportion of claims involve death or brain damage to the infant owing to birth asphyxia and inappropriate deliveries.
- There were incidents due to inadequate fetal monitoring, including care, action taken and the recording of CTGs and pH levels of the fetus leading to delays in instigating treatments and interventions.
- There were delays in performing caesarean sections due to a number of factors including inadequate training and supervision of junior medical staff; inadequately defined chain of command guideline and fear of 'jumping call' in case it upset team working, or allowing arguments to become personal instead of thinking of fetal and maternal well-being; lack of experienced personnel available to perform the emergency operation and lack of theatre facilities or staff to perform the procedure.
- Claims resulted from delays in involving senior medical staff due to fears about not being able to cope or the attitude or inappropriate responses of some seniors.
- Intraoperative problems included equipment failures due to lack of maintenance, training in usage and regular checking of functionality; not always having backup equipment if something malfunctions or is unsafe to use.

- Others included retained products such as placental tissue or swabs and negligent repairs of vaginal, third degree and episiotomy tears.

Gynaecology

In gynaecology features of claims included the following.

- Damage to adjacent organs or vessels during the operation and negligence during the procedure.
- Failed communication and explanations being given to the patient including an inadequate consent process.
- Sterilisation failures due to poor technique and/or inadequate explanation of the risks, alternatives and benefits of the procedure to the patient before the operation.
- Retained swabs, needles and products after surgery without adequate surgical counts and checks on materials used during the procedure.
- Others included failure to diagnose especially around the areas of ectopic pregnancies and ovarian cysts; failure to undertake pregnancy testing before hysterectomies and complications.

Orthopaedics

Orthopaedic claims included the following.

- Retained foreign bodies, diathermy burns and medical errors.
- Operative nerve damage and negligent performance of the procedure.
- Broken or malfunctioning equipment including breaking of drills and screws.
- Missed diagnosis, undiagnosed fractures or delays in diagnosis causing perceived worsening of condition.
- Inadequate consent and communication with the patient to include the risks, alternatives and benefits of treatments and in particular failure to warn the patient of potential complications.
- Postoperative complications such as infections, pressure sores and patient falls.
- Failure to train and supervise juniors appropriately.

Surgical specialities

In surgery claims had the following features.

- Technical errors including patient awareness when the patient is meant to have had a general anaesthetic and poor anaesthetic technique resulting in dental damage.
- Retained foreign bodies including swabs, instruments, blades and needles.
- Diagnostic errors such as missed ectopic pregnancies and appendicitis.
- Postoperative complications often resulting from inadequate explanations given to the patient and a poor consent process.

Accident and emergency

- The vast majority of claims were due to failures in diagnosis and many were related to poor interpretation of X-rays and inappropriate X-rays being requested.
- Failure of training and supervision of junior doctors with an SHO-led service and over 70 per cent of claimants not being seen by a doctor more senior than an SHO.
- About 65 per cent of incidents occurred when there were no middle or senior grade doctors present in the accident and emergency department
- Poor communication and lack of follow-up instructions being given to patients and negative attitudes led patients to take claims further.

The factors which were common across all specialities and emerged from many of the claims included inconsistent and poor record keeping; incomplete or missing documentation especially the most crucial, e.g. CTGs, or investigation results which were claimed to have not been acted upon; inability to locate the staff involved in poor investigation at the time of the incident and no mechanism to track staff down; poor information, communication and consent process leading to dissatisfied and angry patients; unhelpful remarks and attitude problems and inadequate care and attention with poor explanation and no discharge information.

Analysis of these claims helps us to identify the areas where things have the potential to go wrong, where lessons need to be learned to change practices and behaviours and where monitoring systems can be in place for early detection. This would allow for early identification, review and full investigation. They allow for proactive actions to be taken to prevent injuries and untoward outcomes to patients. Examples of good practices implemented as a result include the use of monitors to record the oxygen levels of patients during anaesthesia and the identification of high-risk conditions that patients present with in the accident and emergency department and which need to be assessed by senior doctors. A key component of this approach to effective risk management was instigated by MMI Co. Inc. in the USA through their development and implementation of clinical risk modification programmes[13]. These programmes combine specialty-specific clinical guidelines, monthly reporting of clinical indicators, patients' record review criteria and annual clinical practice surveys in an effort to help providers focus on improving systems and practices that may expose patients to the risk of injuries. MMI's clinical risk modification programmes were developed by national task forces of practising clinicians in consultation with risk management professionals[13]. They are based on frequent analysis of their claims database which helps to identify poor practices and areas of clinical improvement. Based on the information received from their clients, MMI has produced 6-, 8-, 10- and 12-year data summary reports demonstrating that improvements within healthcare systems and clinical practices lead to improved patient outcomes which can have a favourable impact on the frequency and severity of professional liability losses[14]. The experiences of the programme participants also demonstrate changes in practices that take place over time. In the UK and Europe we could learn some lessons from different approaches taken in the USA where risk management practices have been established for much longer. The UK National Framework Document is based on developing indicators for performance, relating inputs, processes and outcomes[15]. Perhaps with cooperation between the professional bodies and the formulation of task forces we could produce the same excellent results.

CONCLUSIONS

The goal of clinical risk modification is to improve the quality of patient care by improving the processes and systems of care and thereby minimise the cost of failures. This chapter has covered much ground in terms of practical tips and experiences to allow readers to act more proactively. Some feel that risk management is a fairly new concept within the UK which is being developed, others would argue we have been doing it for years but the label is new. There are different ways of practising risk management, and thereby fully utilising clinical risk modification strategies, these usually start off in a reactive way and build up to being more proactive and preventative. These are as follows.

Reactive actions for risk modification

- Learning lessons from things that have gone wrong.
- Correction of errors and trying to ensure that they do not happen again.
- Analysis of complaints, near misses, incidents and claims with tracking, trending and sharing of information.
- Management of complaints, near misses, incidents and claims.
- Minimisation of distress and providing support to staff and patients.
- Management of claims.
- Risk containment.
- Risk control.

Proactive actions to risk modification

- Identification of existing risk to ensure that risk awareness and controls are in place.
- Assessment of potential systems failures and making contingency disaster plans.
- Analysis of priorities for action, ongoing review and prioritisation of risks.
- Changes in practices, behaviour and culture of the organisation supported by good change management and organisational development techniques.
- Elimination/reduction of hazards to ensure that risks are controlled, transferred or managed.
- Incorporating quality, risk and audit into one department of clinical effectiveness.

- Use of ICM, MPCs© and working in partnership for seamless, high-quality care demonstrated by standards and outcome measures.
- Addressing clinical effectiveness and patient outcomes to ensure appropriateness of care.

The stage at which you are within your organisation should be easily identifiable and the steps needing to be taken can be learned. One of the most important lessons that healthcare providers can learn is that risk modification is a process not a position. Often staff feel that because they have a risk manager that person has responsibility and accountability for risk, whereas it should be part of everyone's role and responsibility, part of job descriptions and individual objectives. To meet the quality focus and Clinical Governance criteria of the NHS we must practise clinical risk modification through safe and effective practices. The purpose of clinical governance is to ensure healthcare organisations have the right controls, reporting and feedback mechanisms to ensure lessons are learned, performance is measured and that there are clear lines of responsibility and accountability for the overall quality and risk modification of clinical care.

REFERENCES

1. Department of Health (1997) *The New NHS, Modern, Dependable.* Cmnd 3807. HMSO: London.
2. Hickey, J. (1995) The Clinical Negligence Scheme for Trusts. Risk management – a new approach (1). *Clinical Risk*, **1**, (1), 43–46.
3. NHS Executive (1996) *The National Health Service Litigation Authority Framework Document.* 96FP0046. NHS Executive, DOH: Leeds.
4. Carlise, D. (1998) A case for cuts. *Health Management*, **May**, 18–19.
5. Sanderson, I. M. (1998) The CNST: a review of its present function. *Clinical Risk*, **4**, 35–42.
6. Wilson, J. H. (1996) *Integrated Care Management: The Path to Success.* Butterworth-Heinemann: Oxford.
7. Wilson, J. H. (1992) *An Introduction to Multidisciplinary Pathways of Care.* Northern Regional Health Authority, Newcastle upon Tyne.
8. Clinical Negligence Scheme for Trusts (1996) *Risk Management Standards and Procedures: Manual of Guidance.* CNST: Bristol.
9. Heinrich, H. W. and Schaefer, H.-G. (1994) Team performance in the operating room. In *Human Errors in Medicine* (M. S. Bogner ed.). Erlbaum: Hillsdale, NJ.
10. Wilson, J. H. (1997) The Clinical Negligence Scheme for Trusts. *British Journal of Nursing,* **6**, (20), 1166–7.
11. Pincombe, C. (1995) The Clinical Negligence Scheme For Trusts. Risk management – a new approach (2). *Clinical Risk*, **1**, (3), 132–134.
12. March, P. (1995) *Clinical Negligence – Implications for an NHS Trust.* MBA dissertation, Nottingham Trent University.
13. MMI Companies Inc. (1994) *Clinical Risk Modification Programs.* MMI Companies Inc.: Deerfield, IL.
14. MMI Companies Inc. (1991, 1993, 1996) *6, 8, 10 and 12 Year Data Summaries.* MMI Companies Inc.: Deerfield, IL.
15. NHS Executive (1998) *The New NHS, Modern and Dependable: A National Framework for Assessing Performance.* 12394 FPA 5k 2P Feb 98 (RIC). HMSO: London.

4 USING INFORMATION SYSTEMS TO SUPPORT RISK MANAGEMENT

Dennis J. Van Liew

COMPUTERISED INFORMATION AND ANALYSIS FOR RISK MANAGERS

The risk manager's primary goal is to protect the assets of the organisation and to identify high-risk behaviours that could give rise to injury or harm. To perform this role to a high standard, it is essential that the risk manager be able to obtain and analyse information on all aspects of the healthcare organisation systems and processes. The risk manager must determine who is collecting data that could be of use in risk management and who needs access to this data besides those involved in its direct collection.

WHAT INFORMATION DOES THE RISK MANAGER NEED?

Effective identification and assessment of the healthcare organisation's risk exposure is the first step in the risk management process. The risk manager needs data about actual injuries and losses incurred (as discussed previously in Chapters 2 and 3), potential injuries, and data about the overall functioning of systems and processes within the healthcare organisation. This information is frequently found from the following sources:

- Incident reports.
- Complaints.
- Patient records.
- Solicitors' records.
- Policies and procedures.
- Patient and staff satisfaction surveys.
- Clinical audit data, indicators or triggers.
- Maintenance records.
- Verbal reports.
- Training records.

WHO NEEDS TO RECEIVE REPORTS FROM THE RISK MANAGER?

A critical factor in reducing risk is the establishment of an overall feedback loop. Feedback is error driven. Research has shown that feedback delay can have a truly calamitous effect on improving the individual's performance[1]. There are three areas in which feedback can be used to bring errors to people's attention:

- Self-monitoring.
- Environmental error cueing.
- Error discovery by another individual.

A well designed system within a trust should employ all three systems. Finally, it is important to recognise that improving error reporting will take time. MMI Companies, Inc., an international healthcare risk management organisation, has shown that an initial internal training programme will raise reporting and change behaviour somewhat in year one, but it will not be until year three that the great majority of staff will have changed behaviour fully[2].

There are therefore several groups of stakeholders who need feedback; the actual providers of services (clinical and non-clinical), management and the board. Each group needs to have a set of timely reports which identify areas of both potential and actual high risk. These reports need to be further supported by the development of action plans which are designed to help reduce overall risk exposures.

COLLECTION AND ANALYSIS OF DATA

Data collection and analysis is an ongoing process. A recent study undertaken by the Taskforce on Quality in Australian Health Care found a far higher prevalence of admissions associated with an adverse event (16.6 per cent)[3] than the percentage reported by the Harvard study (3.7 per cent)[4]. Commentators have stated that it is difficult to know whether the wide difference is a result of a real gap in the quality of healthcare between the two countries, as there were methodological differences between both studies[5].

In the non-clinical area, a 1996 study done by the UK National Audit Office (NAO) estimated that NHS staff suffered an annual accident rate of 16 accidents per 100 whole-time-equivalent (WTE) staff[6].

Portsmouth Hospitals NHS Trust has established a collection and analysis process for risk data within the hospital which is shown in Figure 4.1. This includes evaluation of the relative risk that each risk event presents to the trust. A key feature of the Portsmouth Hospital approach is weekly, quarterly and trend-driven feedback to local wards and departments.

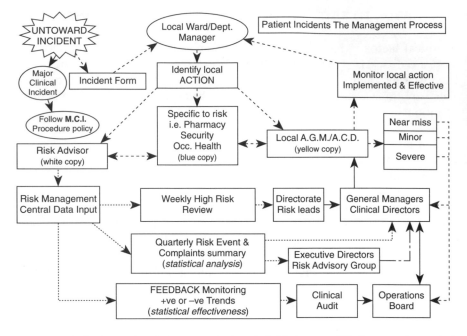

Figure 4.1   Collection and analysis process for hospital risk data. © 1998, Portsmouth Hospitals NHS Trust, reproduced by permission of Phil Hawkins, Corporate Risk Manager.

CHARACTERISTICS OF SUCCESS

A number of key factors can influence whether the risk management department is able successfully to use risk information and technology within the healthcare organisation:

- A clearly defined set of expectations around the use of risk information and technology at the operations level.
- A risk management advisory committee that provides clear guidance with strong participation from both clinical and non-clinical leaders throughout the healthcare organisation.
- A strong total quality management programme focused on maximising the use and return of IT investments.
- A strong customer satisfaction monitoring/management programme.

SYMPTOMS OF COMMON PROBLEMS WITH RISK INFORMATION SYSTEMS

The success of risk information systems in supporting risk management has been mixed. Unless healthcare organisations develop the supporting processes

Table 4.1 Symptoms of common problems with risk information systems

Symptom	Problem
Reports not delivered on time or not delivered with the right type of information.	Lack of control of report preparation and distribution; no formal method for identifying proper report distribution.
Custom report requests for departments/directorates/divisions are lost.	System does not emphasise end user requests. No structure in place to handle requests, operators do not know their system well enough to judge whether requests can be filled and what capabilities are available.
Unusual employee turnover.	Lack of ability of management to retain staff, lack of career development, lack of employee direction by management.
Ongoing differences with vendor regarding contractual obligations and support.	Vendor does not respect staff, inappropriate or weak vendor management, system uses vendor-supplied services poorly.

for ongoing management and effective updating of the risk information system, ensuring quality in data collection processes, and providing for frequent reporting and use in modifying risk behaviours, the risk information system will not be an effective tool.

Systems not fulfilling their potential frequently exhibit the symptoms shown in Table 4.1.

OTHER RISK ANALYSIS TOOLS

In addition to risk reporting systems, there are other information driven tools which a risk manager can use to control exposures. These include benchmarking, comparative clinical indicators, and Multidisciplinary Pathways of Care© (MPCs©) variances[7].

Health and safety benchmarking

Within health and safety, the NAO has identified two areas in which benchmarks can be developed: health and safety incidents, and compliance with health and safety legislation. A few sample benchmarks are as follows:

- Number of staff accidents resulting in injury per 100 WTE staff.
- Number of RIDDOR (Reporting of Injuries, Diseases and Dangerous Occurrences Regulations, 1995) reportable incidents per 100 WTE staff.

- Staff absenteeism rate related to accidents.
- Percentage compliance with health and safety legislation.
- Percentage compliance with manual handling legislation.
- Number of staff personal injury claims per 100 WTE staff.
- The average cost per accident.

For benchmarking to be effective, an agreed common set of definitions must be developed. Once this is accomplished, types and numbers of accidents in similar organisations can be compared to identify strengths and weaknesses, and thereby help all participants to improve. This process can greatly help to reduce the high costs associated with accidents[8].

Clinical risk benchmarking

Within the clinical area, the risk manager must develop a set of clinical indicators for clinical risk benchmarking. Examples of such indicators include:

- General and regional anaesthetic without pulse oximetry in recovery.
- Death or CPR arrest intraprocedurally.
- Antepartum fetal death at > 24 weeks' gestation.
- Neonatal Apgar < 4 at 5 min.
- Patient aged < 24 months with pyrexia, unplanned return to Accident and Emergency within 48 hours.
- Patient left after triage before being seen in Accident and Emergency.
- Inpatient endoscopic surgery procedure resulting in injury to organ.
- Inpatient unplanned return to operating theatre within 48 hours of procedure.
- Inpatient falls that result in patient injury.
- Outpatient pathological fractures (rehabilitation patients).

INCIDENT REPORTING

Incident reporting (as discussed previously in Chapters 2 and 3) is the cornerstone of healthcare risk management. The occurrence of an incident should trigger completion of a report form. Incident report data should be collected and analysed to determine whether there are any trends that represent potential problems in the delivery of care. The results of this analysis should then be distributed and shared with the individuals and departments involved. This should include positive results as well as problem areas.

Definitions

An incident can be defined as any occurrence which is not consistent with the professional standards of care of the patient or the routine operation/policies of the organisation[9].

A near miss is:

> . . . an occurrence which, but for luck or skilful management, would in all probability become an incident[9].

The Concise Oxford Dictionary definition of an incident is:

> . . . an event that is without apparent cause or unexpected: unintentional act, chance, misfortune; including event, especially one causing injury or damage.

H. W. Heinrich's definition of an incident is[10]:

> An uncontrolled and unplanned event in which the action or reaction of an object, substance, person or radiation, results in personal injury or property damage.

The International Labour Office defines an incident as:

> An unexpected, unplanned occurrence which may involve injury.

Lord MacNaughton said:

> An accident is used in the popular and ordinary sense of the word as denoting an unlooked for mishap or an untoward event which is not expected or designed.

Lord Robertson said:

> . . . with regard to legal liabilities, an accident means an unintended and unexpected occurrence which produces error or loss.

Most clinical risk managers consider a clinical error to be any variance from intended treatment, care, therapeutic intention or diagnostic result; there may be untoward outcome or not. Clinical near miss is a clinical error without an untoward outcome. The word error has its roots in Old French or Middle English *errare* meaning to stray, i.e. to err.

Examples of reportable incidents that are more likely to lead to a medicolegal claim

The following is a list of clinical indicators that are associated with a higher likelihood of a potential claim.

- Unexpected or trauma related deaths.
- Brain damage or neurological deficit not present on admission.
- Unexpected amputation due to poor outcome of any procedure/treatment.
- Unplanned removal of organ during surgery.
- More extensive surgery than planned preoperatively.
- Any unplanned return to operating theatre.
- Operations to repair damage due to invasive or endoscopic procedure.
- Failure to act on imaging or pathology result.

- Medication error, including infusion pump problems.
- Hospital incurred trauma.
- Equipment failure leading to patient injury.
- Wrong patient/wrong side – surgery or radiology.
- Self-harm or suicide.
- Complication for which patient was not prepared.
- Misdiagnosis.
- Unplanned admission to ICU/HDU.
- Swab/instrument count incorrect at end of procedure.
- Absent medical notes.
- Hospital incurred trauma.

Source: HRRI, 1996

Models of critical incident reporting

Care givers frequently do not report incidents, let alone near misses. There are many reasons for this. Bark reports on a recent study in North Thames Regional Health Authority, England in which only 54 per cent of house officers discussed their most serious mistake with a senior clinician[11].

Database robustness is directly dependent on the quality of information. The risk manager must therefore take account of the factors required for developing a culture which encourages reporting. These include:

- organisational structures in place – clinical and non-clinical;
- current reporting processes;
- presence of guidelines for preserving report confidentiality;
- current culture (i.e. propensity to report, degree to which organisation is a learning organisation);
- openness to change;
- degree of multidisciplinary working; and
- presence of a board-endorsed risk management strategy.

If these elements are in place, a healthcare organisation can establish an information flow as shown in Figure 4.2. The final output of action feeds directly back to those reporting incidents. This feedback reinforces good behaviour and provides incentives to modify systems and processes to minimise risk.

Incident report design

Incident reports vary in content and structure. Some have only preprinted data elements which can be ticked. Other forms have extensive free text fields. Regardless of form design most reports try capture the following information:

- Name, address and telephone number of individuals involved in incident. For patients and members of staff, patient record numbers, NHS numbers and employee numbers may also be recorded to facilitate later identification.

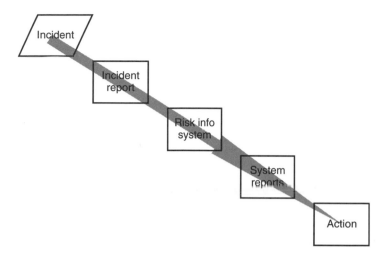

Figure 4.2   Risk information flow in a healthcare organisation.

This information is also helpful in identifying potential claimants and witnesses in cases of litigation.

- Organisation-related information such as admission or incident date, ward/ area involved, discharge diagnosis (e.g. READ or ICD10 code), care givers involved, etc. This can be used as aggregate data to determine whether certain wards, departments or specialties are more 'incident prone'.

- Description of the incident, as well as facts surrounding the event. These may include location of the incident, type of incident (e.g. medication error, slip/trip/fall, lost property, violence to staff), extent of injury incurred, pertinent environmental findings such as position of bed rails, condition of floor, physical defects in equipment, and results of any physical examination to patient, visitor or employee.

The risk manager must balance the goal of designing a simple to use form with the need to collect information about a risk event in order that proper follow up can occur. A example of an incident form is given in Figure 4.3.

LITIGATION MANAGEMENT

Litigation management can be greatly enhanced by the presence of reliable information about all the factors involved in the claim. As many claims are made long after the actual risk event, a fully implemented risk information system can greatly aid the investigation process. Although not quantified, it is also believed that a robust litigation management system can aid the claim manager in ensuring that the claim is processed with a minimum of administrative expense.

PORTSMOUTH HOSPITALS NHS TRUST - ACCIDENT / INCIDENT OR UNEXPLAINED EVENT

To be completed by the member of staff who discovers, witnesses or is notified of the risk event.
Please write in BLOCK CAPITAL LETTERS and tick appropriate boxes as required in black biro pen only.

(if) Patient Hospital No. ....

Person involved Name ....

(if) Staff Personnel No. ....

☐ Male ☐ Female **Age range** ☐ 0–1 months ☐ 1–9 months ☐ 9 months–3.5 years ☐ 3.5 years–16 ☐ 16–60 years ☐ 60+

Incident Date .... Incident Time .... Reported Date ....

Location - Directorate .... Dept/Ward .... Area ....

Category of person:
involved in the incident
i.e. Injured person

☐ Full time employee   ☐ Part time employee   ☐ Contractor   ☐ Agency

☐ Locum   ☐ Volunteer   ☐ Other   ☐ Inpatient

☐ Bank   ☐ Outpatient   ☐ Visitor

People in attendance (please tick one box)

Role - ☐ Attending Nurse ☐ Attending Dr/Consultant ☐ Witness ☐ Other care provider/staff ☐ Other non-care staff

Name .... Address ....

Name .... Address ....

Result of Incident ☐ Fatality ☐ Critical/Severe harm/Damage/Theft   ☐ Minor Harm/Damage/Theft   ☐ Potential Harm/Near Miss
(Fracture/Loss over £1000)   (Bruise/Sprain/Loss under £1000)

If Fatality / Critical follow report system in the front of Risk Event Book

If clinical incident involving patient (tick one box only)

☐ Drug related   ☐ Patients exposure to radiation   ☐ Patient slip/trip/ fall   ☐ Management of medical records   ☐ Medical records contents

☐ Lifting/handling Patients   ☐ Abscondment   ☐ Hospital acquired infection   ☐ Sharps/needle/ patient harm   ☐ Other clinical events

Bed status ....   Medical Equipment Serial Number ....

HAVE YOU COMPLETED YOUR CRITICAL INCIDENT FORM   ☐ Yes   ☐ No   ☐ No form available

If non clinical (tick one box only)

☐ Theft   ☐ Product   ☐ Fire   ☐ Staff lifting/handling   ☐ Hazardous substance

☐ Staff slip/trip/fall/harm   ☐ Road traffic accident   ☐ Contact with electricity   ☐ Struck by moving object   ☐ Staff exposed to radiation

☐ Contact with hot or cold surface   ☐ Vandalism damage   ☐ Accidental   ☐ Equipment   ☐ Self inflicted accident

☐ Staff/Hospital acquired infection   ☐ Gas failure   ☐ Electrical failure   ☐ Medical gases   ☐ Lift failure

☐ Water   ☐ Computer failure   ☐ Physical assault   ☐ Verbal threat   ☐ Damage to property

☐ Clerical error   ☐ Sharps needle sticks - Please notify Occupational Health immediately on Hotline (28) 6478

Description of Injury/ill-health

....
....

Description of what happened FACTS ONLY (include any medication if appropriate)

....
....
....
....
....
....
....
....

Name of examining Doctor ....   Was Doctor informed of incident   YES   NO

Did person receive any attention eg. treatment advice, counselling etc.

☐ None   ☐ First Aid   ☐ A&E   ☐ Doctor   ☐ Occ Health

Details

....
....
....

Date examined .... Time ....

THIS SECTION MUST BE COMPLETED BY WARD MANAGER or CLINICAL MANAGER

Managers comments and action taken FACTS ONLY
What effect has this incident had on:-

1. The member of staff involved - example anticipated days lost due to sickness

....
....

2. Your patient - example as a result of the incident what do you anticipate the increase stay in our care will be - in days

....
....

Causes tick one box   ☐ Staffing level   ☐ Medical grading   ☐ Maintenance   ☐ Human error

☐ Training   ☐ Security   ☐ Procedure error

Was patient's relative informed   ☐ YES   ☐ NO   Date ....

Manager's recommendation to Risk Advisory Group if risk cannot be reduced:

....

Manager's signature ....   Date ....

Check front of book. Does RIDDOR apply?   ☐ YES   ☐ NO

If loss (over £1000) Send BLUE copy to Financial Accountant

WHITE COPY to Risk Manager - YELLOW COPY to AGM - BLUE specific to incident ....
PINK COPY held in Risk Event Book

Risk Management Department (only), please tick this box when entered into CareKey system ☐

If Staff   –   Occupational Health
If Fire   –   Fire Officer
If Security   –   Security Manager

Person completing form .... Signature .... Ext No. ....

Figure 4.3 Sample incident form. © 1998, Portsmouth Hospitals NHS Trust, reproduced by permission of Phil Hawkins, Corporate Risk Manager.

Reporting

The Clinical Negligence Scheme for Trusts defines a claim for clinical negligence as[12]:

> Any demand, however made, but usually by the patient's legal advisor, for monetary compensation in respect of a clinical incident leading to a personal injury.

An essential part of the healthcare organisation's risk management plan should be a system for identifying and reporting actual and potential claims to the risk manager. Both the organisation's form and informal information systems can assist with this task. The risk manager should review all incident reports, internal audit reports, standing committee minutes and other similar documents and follow up where necessary.

The risk manager should also query the complaints system (if not part of an integrated risk information system) for complaints relating to perceived injury or quality of care.

The risk manager must be aware of the requirements for reporting. These vary based upon region and between countries. For example, in England, the CNST has asked English NHS trusts to report all claims once settled including those that are below the trust's excess. There are also requirements for these same trusts to provide quarterly reports above the trust excess.

In addition to reporting, many healthcare organisations are required to provide to their insurer or public body with financial responsibility for payment of claims copies of the following items:

- all expert reports;
- all pleadings including statements/particulars of claim, defence, reply, further and better particulars, interrogatories, etc.;
- relevant witness statements;
- relevant medical records;
- schedules of special damages; and
- counsel's opinions.

Complaint management

To complain means to express dissatisfaction. A complaint is a formal protest. The pressure on the health worker has never been greater and many staff have a deep personal commitment to their job, often above and beyond any reasonable call of duty. When 'things go wrong', staff often feel a sense of failure, regret and disappointment. Many similar feelings are felt by the complainant along with feelings of confusion and anger. It is in both parties' best interest to minimise complaints and resolve those that do arise swiftly and sensitively. (This will be further discussed in Chapters 6 and 7.)

Complaints can be segregated into two categories: informal and formal. An informal complaint, whether by telephone or in person, can, with careful handling, be dealt with rapidly. A formal complaint in the form of a letter, fax or email must usually go through a formal process of review.

The goals of an effective complaint management programme should be as follows:

- There should informal resolution between the complainant and the health-care organisation where possible.
- There should be a complaints procedure separate from the employee grievance procedure.
- There should a formal appeal process.

Information requirements

To improve the complaint management process, there should be a systematic collection of complaints statistics. This should include the number and types of complaints made, the time needed to resolve the complaint, the number of complaint resolutions appealed, the subject of the complaint and the department involved or named in the complainants letter.

Linking complaint data with incidents and litigation

Complaint data are an essential part of an integrated risk information system. The NHS Health Service Commissioner's Annual Report recently released data relating to complaints throughout the UK[13]. His report stated that the NHS established a new unified complaints procedure on 1 April 1996 broadly along the lines recommended in the Wilson Report. (See also Chapters 2, 7 and 8.) 1996–97 showed a record number of complaints made to his office – 2219 complaints, 24 per cent up on the previous year. In addition, the Commissioner processed 2207 items of supplementary correspondence, an increase of 30 per cent. Five major areas were cited by the Health Service Commissioner as opportunities for improvement.

Communication between staff
The importance of communication has now been stressed in the last four annual reports. Examples of poor communication noted in this report include failure to make sure all information relevant to a patient's care was recorded and passed on where appropriate; failure adequately to communicate hospital policies and procedures to staff and to ensure that systems were modified to meet new policies; and failure to record community health visits in the patient record.

Record keeping
Poor record keeping continues to cause complaints. A specific example identified deficiencies in one trust's policy on access and amendment to patient records.

Communication with relatives of dead or dying patients

Failures in communication can compound the distress of relatives of patients who are dying or have died. One example cited is the failure to console a daughter whose father had died the night before. The problem was further compounded by failing to respond to the subsequent complaint and then responding with a letter containing several errors.

Mortuary and post mortem procedures

Problems concerning mortuary arrangements also were cited, including a doctor's lack of awareness of the procedure for requesting a post mortem.

Complaint handling

A large number of complaints are received by the Commissioner relating to the handling of the original complaint. Lack of awareness about local complaint-handling procedures, incorrect sequencing, confusion about when a case can be referred to independent professional review, fuzzy timescales, and lack of independent monitoring of complaints handling (including observance of time-scales and accuracy of replies) were all cited as examples.

A relatively recent phenomenon reported informally by a number of trusts is the use of the complaints process by solicitors to test the system before entering the legal process. Trusts need to make sure, therefore, that the complaints process is fully integrated into the risk information management process and not compartmentalised because of fears of the sensitive nature of the information being collected.

Mike Surkitt-Parr at Leicester General Hospital NHS Trust has proposed that a well-managed complaints process using an integrated risk information system can be an effective way of reducing the incidence of claims[14]. This integration can also serve to show staff the benefits of meeting complainants' needs early on by making and maintaining early contact.

The challenge to meet needs will surely increase as patients become more knowledgeable and assertive about their rights of access to various treatment options. The opportunity to register a complaint is now easier too. For example, the Health Service Commissioner has put a Complaint Form on the Internet (*see http://health.ombudsman.org.uk/form/healthfm.htm*). Therefore, it is critical for the NHS constantly to improve not only the handling of complaints, but also their prevention.

INFORMATION FLOWS

A major task of risk managers is to determine the appropriate risk information system for their healthcare organisation. This system needs to support a variety of risk information tasks and have the ability to be accessed by a number of staff throughout the organisation.

A first step in system selection is identification of current and future risk information flows. These can be captured through use of an audit tool which can then serve as part of an evaluation form when reviewing commercial systems.

Table 4.2 provides an overview of the items which need to be reviewed.

Table 4.2 Items to consider when commissioning a risk information system

Functional requirement	Essential/ desirable
Incident reporting	
Incident date, time, specific location, consultant responsible, patient status (inpatient/outpatient/day case), admission diagnosis and incident description.	Essential
Injury details and follow-up treatment, incident severity.	Essential
Lost work days (if employee).	Essential
Equipment involved details.	Essential
Recording of actions taken after incident, including witness details.	Essential
Persons notified and individual reporting incident.	Essential
Complaints	
Patient's name, hospital number, date of birth and address.	Essential
Complainant details.	Essential
Response logging, including dates.	Essential
Allows details recorded of decisions taken.	Essential
Litigation	
Automatic data transfer to/from other risk information system module including incident reporting and complaint management.	Essential
Recording of plaintiff and defendant solicitor details and costs.	Essential
Stage-of-claim reporting.	Essential
Third party financial reporting to external organisations whether public sector of commercial.	Essential
Recording of patient notes and X-rays.	Desirable
Correspondence	
Data merging from database into standard format letters.	Essential
Reports	Essential
Risk summaries covering all incidents, complaints and litigation relating to a specific location in the hospital by any field.	
Incident/complaint/litigation statistical reports by specific location, department and site.	Essential
Ad hoc reports as required.	Essential

Software – integrated systems and interfaces

An integrated system is one in which all data from the various risk information software applications and modules reside in a single database, accessible via all system terminals. There are commercial systems available which offer an integrated solution that may meet all the organisations needs. Alternatively, there are other systems, each with its own database, connected to one another by specialised software called *interfaces*. The main purpose of an interface is to make a system look integrated to the end user. Interfaces are 'gateways' that allow systems to interact and appear integrated, and, like any piece of software, interfaces have to be designed, maintained and upgraded.

Client/server and database technology

New generation risk management information systems are now becoming available employing client/server technology. Client/server technology allows computer users to take advantage of increased speed and processing power by distributing computing activities across a network of interconnected computers. Client/server architecture allows the distribution of data processing, storage, retrieval and presentation across multiple powerful servers, data repositories and end-user PCs or workstations.

For the risk manager, this allows many new opportunities, including collection of incidents at ward or department level by having staff key reporting

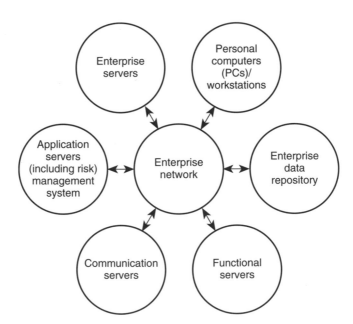

Figure 4.4   Risk information system network.

directly into the network. Department managers and clinical directors can now query their own data locally without having to ask the risk management department to prepare a report. These systems also employ email which means that risk alert bulletins can be sent quickly to staff throughout the organisation.

With client/server technology, risk information can truly become integrated, see Figure 4.4.

Specifications

The risk manager must make sure that the system selected will run on the healthcare organisation network and PC. Software vendors can provide the system requirement specifications. It is also wise that the risk manager ask for a minimum of three referees including a organisation where a site visit is possible.

In addition to these general requirements, specific requirements are also recommended, as shown in Table 4.3.

Support services

Some software vendors offer extensive after-sales support, while others operate just a telephone help desk. The risk manager must identify those services the healthcare organisation needs which are not readily available in-house. A list of services is provided in Table 4.4.

Internet and intranets

The internet offers risk managers the chance for collaborative access to risk data. Not only can data be shared, but new programmes and risk audit tools can broadly be accessed by the healthcare organisation, without the need to install individual copies of software on each user's desktop computer. The new systems will accessible through a broad variety of computer operating systems, including Windows 3.1, Windows 95, Windows 98, Windows NT, UNIX, and Macintosh. Increasingly, any computing environment will support use of a 'Web Browser'.

The power of the browser is that, once installed on a computer for one purpose, it can be used for many other purposes, including access to a broad range of applications, including four kinds of media that previously were accessible only in three totally separate environments:

- text, such as risk management manuals and reference materials;
- software, such as claims management software;
- multimedia, such as training videos or videos showing details of key locations, equipment, or manufacturing processes; and
- risk manager discussion forums.

Table 4.3 Specific requirements for risk information software

Functional requirement	Essential/ desirable
General system requirements Compatible with Microsoft Windows and OS2 platforms.	Essential
Allows GUI using multiple screens.	Essential
Allows data downloading from other systems.	Essential
Ability to select records on user-defined basis.	Essential
Allows data to be driven by user-defined code tables.	Essential
Allows for audit facilities.	Essential
Documentation provided on all database files on system.	Essential
Documentation provided on upgrades including actions required by users.	Essential
Screen painting/editing facilities available for user defined fields, field lengths, screen formats menus and which data items are mandatory.	Desirable
Allows data to be uploaded to database from other systems.	Desirable
Each item of data is required to be input only once.	Essential
User may redefine existing and add new validation/integrity checks to prevent data inconsistency.	Desirable
System contains context sensitive, on-line, and user-defined help.	Desirable
Report generator User friendly *ad hoc* reporting is available.	Essential
Operational Full unattended backup of entire system.	Essential
Software/hardware resilience built into the system.	Essential
Formal disaster recovery procedure in place.	Essential
Formal development strategy for the proposed system including development tools used, post-implementation enhancement procedures, and frequency of upgrades.	Essential
System characteristics Average and maximum response times to enter a complete incident on a database of 4000–10 000 records.	Essential
Average and maximum response times to perform the following on a database of 4000–10 000 records to: log on system, move between menus, create passwords, and print reports.	Essential
Application security Unique identifier for each user.	Essential
User profiles, user activity logs, and user access privilege reports.	Essential

Table 4.4 Support services for risk information software

Functional requirement	Essential/ desirable
Project management services including implementation project plan, user trial and acceptance testing.	Optional
Training Details of the consultancy included at the time of implementation.	Desirable
Details of the ongoing consultancy support.	Desirable
Technical/user support including service level agreement defining:	Essential
(a) User assistance available.	Essential
(b) Procedure for requesting assistance with guaranteed response times.	Essential
(c) Escalation procedures.	Essential
(d) Change request procedures.	Essential
(e) Fault correction procedure with an agreed priority system.	Essential
(f) The availability of training courses after implementation.	Essential
Maintenance including software upgrades and new software releases.	Essential
Documentation provided including user guides, technical system specifications, and reference guides. Procedure for documentation upgrades.	Essential

Useful web sites

The number of web sites continues to multiply daily. The following sites currently represent a selection of some of the most useful sites for risk managers, particularly clinical risk managers. The list is not comprehensive.

- Evidence-based practice on the internet (e.g. Cochrane databases): (http://www.shef.ac.uk/uni/academic/R-Z/scharr/ir/netting.html).
- American Society for Healthcare Risk Management: (http://www.ashrm.org).
- MMI Companies, Healthcare Risk Management Source: (http://www.mmicompanies.com).
- Healthcare Risk Resources International: (http://www.hrri-mmi.com).
- Health and Safety at Work (Ireland): (http://www.hsa.ie/osh/welcome.htm).
- Health and Safety Promotion in the European Union: (http://www.hsa.ie/osh/europrog.htm).
- Health and Safety Executive (HSE), UK: (http://www.open.gov.uk/hse/hsehome.htm).
- Institute of Occupational Safety and Health (IOSH): (http://www.iosh.co.uk/).
- European Agency for Health and Safety at Work: (http://www.eu-osha.es/).

- WorkSafe Western Australia: (http://www.wt.com.au/safetyline/index.html).
- Harvard Risk Management Foundation (HRM): (http://www.rmf.org/).
- The British Healthcare Internet Association: (http://www.bhia.org/).
- Risk World: (http://www.riskworld.com/).
- Loughborough University Centre for Hazard and Risk Management: (http://www.loughborough.ac.uk/departments/bs/excharm.html).
- National Health Service (NHS) Information Management and Technology (IMT) within the UK: (http://www.imt4nhs.exec.nhs.uk/ctf.html).
- NHS Executive: Controls Assurance (http://www.open.gov.uk/doh/riskman.html).

BENEFITS IDENTIFICATION

The procurement of a risk information system must usually be supported by a business case. A key element of this is benefits identification. These benefits can usually be found in the following categories: cash releasing benefits including reductions in data management time and claim administration costs; improvements in the quality of care; efficiency benefits; organisation-related and supplier-related benefits.

CONCLUSIONS

A key element in the provision of risk management is a fully integrated risk information system. These systems help the risk manager manage daily tasks, analyse trends and provide feedback to the organisation and external organisations as required. The rise of both client/server networks and the internet/intranets means that risk managers will be able to begin to benchmark their organisation and share information in novel ways.

REFERENCES

1. Reason, J. (1990) *Human Error*. Cambridge University Press: Cambridge.
2. MMI Co. (1996) *10 Year Data Summary*. MMI Co.: Deerfield, IL.
3. Australian Health Minister's Advisory Council (1996) *The Final Report of the Taskforce on Quality in Australian Health Care*. Australian Health Minister's Advisory Council.
4. Brennan, T. A., Leape, L. L., Laird, N. M. *et al.* (1991) The nature of adverse events in hospitalised patients – results of the Harvard Medical Practice Study II. *New England Journal of Medicine*, **324,** 377–384.
5. Buchan, H. and Brook, C. (1997) Quality in Australian hospitals – who cares? *International Journal for Quality in Healthcare*, **9,** 243–244.
6. National Audit Office (1996) *Health and Safety in NHS Acute Trusts in England*. National Audit Office: London.
7. Wilson, J. H. (1996) *Integrated Care Management: The Path to Success?* Butterworth-Heinemann: Oxford.

8. Health and Safety Executive (1993) *The Cost of Accidents and Work*. Health and Safety Guidance Series. Health and Safety Executive.
9. Wilson, J. H. (1998) Incident reporting. *British Journal of Nursing*, **7**, (11), 670–671.
10. Heinrich, H. W. and Schaefer, H.-G. (1994) Team performance in the operating room. In *Human Errors in Medicine* (M. S. Bogner ed.). Erlbaum: Hillsdale, NJ.
11. Bark, P. (1997) Human factors analysis – reducing the culture of blame. *Healthcare Risk Resource*, **1**, (3), 2–3.
12. Clinical Negligence Scheme for Trusts (1996) *Data Collection and Claim Assessment Procedures*. NHS Litigation Authority: London.
13. Health Service Commissioner (1997) *Annual Report 1996–97*. HMSO: London.
14. Surkitt-Parr, M. (1998) Can good complaints handling reduce the incidents of claims? *Healthcare Risk Resource*, **1**, (4), 6–7.

5 CLINICAL RISK IN PRIMARY CARE

Thoreya Swage

INTRODUCTION

When the National Health Service (NHS) came into existence on 5 July 1948, Britain was provided with a comprehensive healthcare system which was free at the point of delivery to those who needed it regardless of income or advantage. The young NHS, while bringing together private and voluntary hospitals under a unitary system, was, however, a compromise from the start and this was particularly so with the community and primary care services. Community services (e.g. district nurses and health visitors) remained a local authority responsibility until 1974 and primary care providers, general practitioners (GPs), dentists, high street pharmacists and opticians (optometrists) stayed outside the nationalised service, being self-employed contractors to the NHS.

As a consequence the primary care practitioners were very much left alone to develop their services in the community. The negotiated national contracts under which they provided their services were then not significantly modified for over the next forty years. This situation changed dramatically during the late 1980s when the government undertook to review the NHS, principally the hospital, community and mental health services, which set off ripples in the remainder of the healthcare sector[1, 2]. With the changes came an increase in the expectation of the general public to have the best in healthcare and, when this did not occur, complaints and litigation soared manifesting mostly in the acute sector in high-risk specialties such as obstetrics and anaesthesia.

In primary care, however, such considerations were not thought to be of great importance as clinical risk was less of a threat, any financial risk to the individual business was not a problem as the state provided the bulk of an individual practitioner's income, and public expectation of the standards of service in this arena was relatively low.

In 1989, this began to change when free eye tests and dental check-ups were abolished for the general public (except for exempt groups). Optometrists and general dental practitioners were then obliged to begin to seek income from the private sector as the public were unwilling to pay for what were hitherto 'free goods'.

Further changes were to follow with the new general practitioner (GP) contract[3] and dental contract in 1990 specifying the delivery of particular

Table 5.1   Key NHS milestones in primary care

1948	Inception of the NHS and family doctors agree to enter into contract with the NHS
1989	Free eye tests and dental check-ups abolished (except exempt groups)
1990	GP Contract and Dental Contract
1991	Purchaser/provider split and GP fundholding
1992	*Fundamental review of dental remuneration*
1994	GP fundholding accountability framework and the concept of a primary-care led NHS
1994	*Improving NHS Dentistry* – Green Paper
1995	Total fundholding
1996	*Primary Care: The Future* *Choice and Opportunity* *Delivering the Future* *Pharmacy in the New Age*
1997	*The New NHS, Modern, Dependable* – abolishing fundholding in 1999
1998	GP commissioning groups Personal Medical Services Pilots Personal Dental Services Pilots
1999	Primary care groups including primary care trusts Clinical governance

clinical services and, in 1991, the establishment of the purchaser/provider split[2] involving GPs in the new role of purchasing healthcare on behalf of their local populations. Initially, this new role was as GP fundholders responsible for their own budget to buy specific elements of healthcare for their practice population. With the change in government in 1997, all GPs were required to be involved in such activities as part of new bodies called primary care groups and the remit widened to the purchasing of all healthcare[4]. See Table 5.1.

This clearly meant new risks and new accountabilities. For the six years of fundholding, accountability was brought together formally with the GP fund-holder accountability framework[5] in 1994. This covered management and financial responsibilities as well as professional and public accountabilities. Primary care groups are expected to follow a similar process in setting up their accountability mechanisms for the spending of public money[6]. This chapter will build upon in greater detail the issues discussed in Chapter 1.

WHO'S IN PRIMARY CARE?

In general, primary care health professionals perform their work in the community, in or close to patients' homes, ensuring that the health services the public require are available and accessible. Primary care is provided by:

- general medical practitioners and their healthcare teams;
- general dental practitioners;
- community pharmacists;
- high street opticians (optometrists);
- community and mental health staff working in the community setting;
- social services; and
- the independent sector, e.g. nursing and residential homes, charitable institutions, patient organisations and so on.

There is a close link between health and social care, as often one merges into the other in terms of patient needs, and this has been recognised by the requirement that primary care groups work with social services in the planning, commissioning and provision of community health services.

For the purposes of this chapter, however, only the risks applicable to the independent contractors will be considered (i.e. GPs, dentists, high street pharmacists and optometrists or opticians).

WHAT RISKS ARE IN PRIMARY CARE?

The concept of a primary-care led NHS has recognised the need for greater integration and development of primary healthcare services, in particular, bringing together those professionals who, although they may be close geographically, have tended to continue their services with little communication amongst themselves, e.g. general practitioners and community pharmacists.

However, by far the greatest emphasis is on the development of GP services and the primary healthcare team. There is no single agreed definition of the primary healthcare team although it is generally understood to be those health professionals working in and around a practice, with the GP and the core team (administrative staff and practice nurse) at its centre.

GPs are beginning to recognise that the risks, in general, in primary care are wide ranging and too important to ignore. This is particularly so as the volume of work is increasing, the demands of patients become more pressing and with the continued inexorable shift of clinical work from the secondary sector to the community.

Clinical risk cannot be seen in isolation of the other risks primary care practitioners face as many processes are interconnected and impact upon each other. The risks in primary care can be divided into risks relating to the business of the individual practitioner, clinical risk and risks as a purchaser of other health services.

Risks as a business

General practitioners are independent contractors: they are not employees of the NHS. They are, however, dependent on the NHS if they are to provide (and to be paid for) NHS services. A GP has to apply to the local health authority to provide NHS services and appear on the medical list for that area, otherwise payment for those services would not be forthcoming.

Risk management can be defined as the identification, analysis and economic control of those risks which can threaten the assets or the earning capacity of an enterprise. Nowhere is this more true than in general practice. GPs are responsible for providing the physical environment, the staff and the equipment as part of their services to the public. If the environment is not conducive to good clinical care then the risk of things going wrong increases. This can pose quite a burden on individual practitioners although help is at hand from the NHS.

Practice premises
The biggest challenge for new general practitioners (if they are to be a partner) is to buy into the practice and share the financial burden of the cost of running the business; the largest expenditure of which is the fabric of the building, the surgery premises. The Statement of Fees and Allowances (SFA) provides some support in the guise of cost rent schemes (essentially interest-free loans) for building new surgeries and improvement grants (actual financial grants) for extensions and other such upgrades for existing surgeries, but GPs still have to contribute the bulk of the funds to make up the full cost of each project[7]. Strict criteria have been set in the SFA and the money is only forthcoming from the NHS if these are met. Furthermore, the SFA have not kept pace with the changes in primary care in recent years, i.e. the need to have extra space in the GP surgery for the wider primary healthcare team e.g. community mental health teams, professions allied to medicine and so on. Flexibility in this area was introduced by the White Paper *Delivering the Future* in updating some of the cost rent schedules and loans and grants for GPs to buy out of leases on sub-standard premises[8].

There is a need to balance the requirements of patient confidentiality during consultations, the security of practice staff and of clinical records with reasonable accessibility to the GP and other clinical staff in the structure and integrity of the surgery premises. Poor adherence to these criteria can have serious consequences such as vulnerability of practice staff to violent patients or a breach of confidentiality of patient information.

Information technology systems
As primary care has grown so have the information technology systems to support it, both in complexity and cost. There are, for example, clinical and 'purchasing' (fundholding and successor) systems within the practice and between the practice and other organisations. The latter include the GP links between the practice and the health authority to ensure the electronic transfer of information on patient data and registration and 'items of service' data (claims for specific GP services carried out in the practice such as immunisations and vaccinations and so on). There are also links between practices

and hospitals for the transfer of clinical information e.g. pathology results. This has been brought together in the NHS Net, a secure IT system within the wider internet.

Here confidentiality of patient information is of paramount importance and of potentially greatest risk in terms of who within a practice has access to this information and who else sees this data on its journey through the IT system. Consideration needs to be given to the organisation of the backup process if the IT system suddenly crashes and the subsequent difficulty of obtaining patient data when required. The greatest risk, yet to be tested, is when the year 2000 arrives and some call/recall and appointment systems which are dependent on computers, which do not recognise the turn of the century, fail. This could cause chaos both administratively and clinically particularly if breast screening and cervical cytology screening call/recall systems go awry and some potential cancers are missed. In addition, patients may be deleted from the practice systems if their date of birth is no longer recognised and so will not have access to the care they require, e.g. over-75 checks. This eventuality has, in some part, been recognised and extra funding has been made available by the government to update such computers.

The millennium problem aside, another area of risk is the substantial amount of money required for purchasing appropriate IT systems, maintenance and upgrades. The SFA provides for a relatively small contribution to the capital and maintenance costs of computer systems in general practice but the bulk of the financial burden falls to the GPs. This is another difficulty with the SFA as it currently stands. Careful risk assessment needs to be made during the process of investing large sums of money in computerisation and where failures/theft/damage can dramatically impair the functioning of the practice.

The White Papers, *Primary Care: The Future; Choice and Opportunity*[9] and *Primary Care: Delivering the Future*[8] have outlined the availability of incentives to encourage GP practices to join the NHS Network and to reduce the risk of buying a poor IT system by proposing a link between reimbursement and accredited computing systems.

Human resources

It is clear that the increased emphasis on developing primary care in recent years has taken its toll on recruitment and retention of GP partners and practice staff. The Medical Practices Committee Survey (1996) revealed that the total number of applications per vacancy was 9.1 in 1995 as opposed to 13.8 in 1994, the biggest reduction being the number of applications by men[10]. The majority of applicants for part-time jobs were women. Comments were noted on the unwillingness of applicants to be flexible in their choice of working hours and commitment to the practice. The length of time to fill a vacancy was prolonged in 1995: it took approximately nine months to fill just under 80 per cent of vacancies compared to six months in the previous year. The main reason for GPs leaving the NHS was to retire (most taking early retirement at the age of 60), the second most important reason was to take other GP posts and other posts in the NHS. Clearly, this represents a greater stress, hence risks, on the remaining GPs in practice to manage personnel changes within a surgery as well as maintaining and developing services.

The change in the rules for the out of hours responsibility has, to some extent, alleviated the 24 hour care requirement on individual GPs. No longer is the GP principal held responsible for the actions of the doctor on call and the burden can be shared with local colleagues in the form of GP cooperatives. In addition, the need for home visits could be reduced by patients attending 'out of hours primary care centres' where the GPs are in a relatively safe environment should they have to deal with potentially violent patients.

However, cooperatives have developed more rapidly than the quality control systems required to ensure that the best level of care to patients is maintained. For example, the use of telephone advice and nurse practitioners instead of actual home visits may put the responsible GP at greater risk professionally if there are no guidelines or protocols to support this method of working.

It is well recognised that, for a GP, difficulties with partnership agreements and disputes can be extremely stressful as well as financially draining for those concerned. It is particularly difficult for the GP or GPs that leave a partnership. They may have invested much money into the practice premises which they may have to relinquish if they were to move out. This is disruptive to the patients of the troubled practice who may be uncertain as to whom to go with should the partnership split. As the number of patients on a GP's list is important to the income of the GP this could have a devastating effect on the practice finances if there were to be mass changes in the patient population. Furthermore, additional financial investment would be required if a new practice were to be formed and, although some support is available from the health authority, this represents considerable financial risk to the individual practitioner.

Once a new GP principal is appointed, the next step is to negotiate the investment required of the new partner by the practice to take on some of the financial burden and hence the practice profits. An essential aspect of this agreement is to have clarity on the time period it would take for the new partner to reach parity, i.e. have an equal share of the income arising from the patients on the list and therefore, the practice profits. If this is not set down as a legal agreement then the new partner is at risk of losing out on a fair share of the practice income.

GPs, as employers of their practice staff, are charged with the responsibility for ensuring that they are appropriately trained to perform their tasks. This can be a real problem for employees, particularly for practice nurses. Although nurses are required to update their professional knowledge as part of their continuing education, the ease by which this is achieved is dependent on the willingness of the employing GP to release the nurse for training. The 'risk' of losing income by allowing the nurse to go on training courses needs to be balanced by the potential clinical risk of poor practice.

Similarly, the training needs of the administrative staff (e.g. practice managers and reception staff) should be considered alongside the needs and risks of the business.

As more is demanded of primary care and new types of specialist nurses come onto the scene who are able to manage and prescribe for chronic conditions, the need for integrated care management and multidisciplinary working becomes increasingly urgent. This system of working has been well developed in the hospital sector and is beginning to appear in the GP surgery[11].

Clinical risks

The 1990 GP terms and conditions of service were introduced after concern over inconsistent care provided to the public due to poor definition of the type of service GPs were required to provide to patients on their list. The general medical services were tightened up albeit in the wake of much opposition by the GP bodies and have survived so far with little modification. This is certain to change after the evaluation of the Primary Care Act pilot schemes in which a whole practice can undertake to provide personal medical services similar to general medical services[12]. In addition to the basic general medical services, a GP can also offer other clinics in the surgery, provided certain criteria are satisfied, which cover coronary heart disease prevention and chronic diseases such as asthma and diabetes. Although this is usually delegated to the practice nurse or health visitor, the GP is still responsible for ensuring that the nurse is appropriately qualified to perform such a task. See Table 5.2.

Table 5.2 GP terms and conditions of service

A doctor shall render to his patients:

- 'All necessary and appropriate personal medical services of the type usually provided by General Medical Practitioners.'
- Advice on general health including the significance of diet, exercise, the use of tobacco, the consumption of alcohol and the misuse of drugs or solvents.
- A physical examination, where appropriate.
- Where appropriate, vaccination or immunisation against measles, mumps, rubella, pertussis, poliomyelitis, diphtheria and tetanus.
- Referral, where appropriate, to other NHS services and social services.
- Health checks to over 75-year-olds on their list on an annual basis.

Optional services:

- Child health surveillance
- Minor surgery
- Contraceptive services
- Maternity (obstetric) services

The blurred boundaries between primary and secondary care
The background against which the General Medical Services have developed since 1990, however, has not remained constant. With the development of fundholding and the subsequent greater involvement of GPs in primary care groups, the boundaries between primary and secondary care have become more blurred. This may have been acceptable to those practitioners who wished to push back the frontiers of primary care, however, greater clinical risks were exposed as the methods of monitoring the quality of care provided by the new processes did not keep up with the speed of development of the innovations.

NHS trusts, with ever greater pressure to save money, began to modify their services to their benefit without much consideration of the general practitioner, for example, inpatient elective surgery was soon shifted to day cases. This shortened the length of stay of patients in hospital, hence providing a cheaper service, but increased the burden of the GP in terms of immediate management for possible complications and follow up in the community. This posed a great clinical risk as GPs felt ill equipped to look after patients with conditions in which they had little or no training.

Another example is the request from hospital clinicians for GPs to prescribe expensive drugs about which the GP has very little knowledge or expertise, e.g. erythropoietin for renal replacement therapy, or cytotoxic drugs. This can relieve the hospital drug budget but places pressure on the GP prescribing budgets. A third area is the requirement for some clinical services to be performed in the community, e.g. anticoagulation clinics, without any extra resources to support the GP.

All of these examples raise the issues of which services are 'core' as opposed to 'non-core' in primary care, clinical responsibility, appropriate training and resources. Many of these matters have been picked up by the General Medical Services Committee of the British Medical Association in the document stating the BMA's stance on the issue[13]. The debate still continues and will probably develop further as the primary care groups are established from April 1999 and beyond. Some practitioners have taken local initiatives and have negotiated agreements whereby a trust is required to consult with GPs and, if appropriate, identify resources to support the change, before implementing a service modification which would affect primary care.

The prescribing budget
One of the increasing key areas of concern for practices has been the management of the prescribing budget and the clinical dilemmas which can arise. This budget, which in the past has been allocated to fundholding practices only, is for all the drugs prescribed in the GP surgery. Non-fundholders have had indicative budgets only. Although no patient should be denied any medication that is clinically indicated, there is great pressure for practices to achieve the best value for money by using techniques such as generic prescribing and drug formularies together with medical and prescribing advice from the local

health authority. As with any budget that is overspent one year, the following year's budget is used to cover this problem leaving a resulting smaller budget for that year.

The other great pressure on the prescribing budget is the constant introduction of new and expensive drugs into the NHS which may or may not be more effective in treating people and, if they are marketed well, can raise patient expectation (and therefore demand) for these drugs. Decisions then have to be taken as to which drug treatments should be given with associated clinical risks of not prescribing other treatments.

With the establishment of primary care groups every practice will have to hold a prescribing budget and tackle these difficult issues.

The development of nurse prescribing, after many years of being piloted, is to be extended to enable all appropriately qualified district nurses and health visitors to participate[14]. This initiative could help to achieve some consistency of prescribing, as this process would be guided by appropriate formularies and prescribing protocols. The mechanism by which this could be achieved would be through specific nurse-led clinics in the primary care setting.

The need for continuous professional training of GPs has been recognised nationally by the Royal College of General Practitioners (RCGP) and the General Medical Council (GMC) and systems such as accreditation are being debated and discussed. The GMC has produced a guide for the standards expected of a doctor which sets out the basic principles of good practice recognising the need to 'keep professional knowledge and skills up to date' and to 'work with colleagues in the ways that best serve patients' interests'[15]. Performance assessors with medical and non-clinical backgrounds are part of the mechanism to ensure that these standards are met and that risk to the general public by practitioners who are not fit to practise are minimised.

Clinical governance
As previously discussed in Chapter 1, The White Paper, *The New NHS, Modern, Dependable*, introduced a new statutory duty on NHS trusts of clinical governance. From April 1999 (subject to legislation), the process of clinical governance will place a duty on all health professionals to ensure that the level of clinical service they deliver to patients is 'satisfactory, consistent and responsive'[4]. Table 5.3 shows the characteristics of a quality organisation, as described in the White Paper.

This is of concern to primary care as the fourth level of primary care groups (the primary care trusts) will be subject to this statutory duty. Clinical risk, adverse incidents and poor clinical performance feature clearly in the areas to be covered by clinical governance and will require further work and development in this sector of healthcare.

Clinical audit
Clinical audit, an area which has been developed in primary care, is a mechanism whereby clinicians can examine their practice and improve not only their

---

Table 5.3 Characteristics of a quality organisation (reproduced from *The New NHS, Modern, Dependable* 1997)

- Quality improvement processes in place, e.g. clinical audit, and integrated with the quality programme for the whole organisation.
- Leadership skills developed at clinical team level.
- Evidence-based practice in day-to-day use with infrastructure to support it.
- Good practice, ideas and innovations (which have been evaluated) systematically disseminated within and outside the organisation.
- Clinical risk reduction programmes in place.
- Incidents detected and openly investigated and lessons promptly applied.
- Lessons for clinical practice systematically learned from complaints made by patients.
- Problems of poor clinical performance recognised at an early stage and dealt with to prevent harm to patients.
- All professional development programmes reflect the principles of clinical governance.
- The quality of data collected to monitor clinical care is itself of a high standard.

---

services but also outcomes for patients. Increasingly, audit has become a multi-disciplinary process such as through the use of integrated care pathways reflecting the fact that care for the patient is provided by a number of different health professionals and in different settings across the primary/secondary interface. This is a system whereby such a multidisciplinary setting in primary care can reveal where there are deficiencies in the processes of care and, hence, areas of risk, which can be addressed.

Vigilance is required particularly with the greater emphasis on multidisciplinary working. This situation may provide an excuse for a health professional not to take on responsibility for the care of an individual patient or, conversely, health professionals may work beyond their professional competence if, for example, a nurse prescribes a drug ignoring an agreed protocol[16], or advice is given by a community pharmacist to a GP on a prescribing issue for which the pharmacist has little knowledge.

Another area is the complaints process, which, whilst potentially threatening to the health professional, is a means of identifying risk through immediate feedback by the users of primary care services. The new procedure introduced in 1996 simplified the process[17] and has ensured that complaints are dealt with swiftly and promptly, reducing the risk of escalation and possible litigation through misunderstanding, that ultimately could severely damage the reputation of the clinician concerned.

Risks as a purchaser

The introduction of the GP as a commissioner and provider of health services has opened up a number of challenges, and with them, risks. Within a finite resource decisions have to be made to commission the best value available care for a local population. This is an area of development which has continued to change since the introduction of the concept of the GP as a purchaser of health-care. Initially, this was through the establishment of fundholding and has now developed into a number of models including GP commissioning groups[18], personal medical services pilots[11] and primary care groups[4], as set out in Table 5.4.

The demands of patients and the fast pace of development of new drugs and medical technologies have often outstripped the capacity of healthcare

Table 5.4 Summary of characteristics of GP commissioning groups, personal medical services pilots and primary care groups

	GP commissioning groups	Personal medical services pilots	Primary care groups
Population covered	Up to 100 000	Up to 100 000	Typically 100 000
Budget	Prescribing budget for general practice. GP fundholder budget. May have indicative HCHS budget.	General medical services. Some of the HCHS budget as negotiated.	Hospital and community health services (HCHS). Prescribing budget for general practice. General medical services budget.
Function	Purchasing fundholding procedures. General practice prescribing.	Provision of personal medical services (PMS), three categories: salaried GP schemes, practice-based contracts for PMS, practice based contracts for PMS + some HCHS.	Purchasing all healthcare on behalf of their population.
Other characteristics			Four levels: advisory, devolved budget, standing body, primary care trust including provision of community health services.
Time period	Two-year pilot.	Three-year pilot.	All practices to be part of a PCG by April 1999.

purchasers to buy them. This then poses difficult questions for purchasers to decide who and what healthcare patients would be entitled to.

The options

Two options are then available: one is to purchase more than can be afforded and the other is not to buy services that are considered to be lower on the list of priorities.

The first option results in an overspend which then has to be recovered through the slowing down of the use of health services, e.g. longer waiting times for operations, spending savings made elsewhere in the system, or using the budget for the following year as a first call. Each of the courses of action pose a potential clinical risk to the patients concerned if they do not have timely access to the treatment they require.

The second course of action is not to purchase some services at all, ideally those that are deemed not clinically necessary, e.g. cosmetic surgery. However, there are always clinical arguments for those patients whose need is for an 'unnecessary' procedure. Either way this, too, presents a potential clinical risk.

Clinical effectiveness

One process that is growing in momentum in relation to quality and risk is the development of clinical effectiveness and the use of this to inform healthcare decisions. Clinical effectiveness is a complex process; however, it has four main elements including research, dissemination of the evidence, implementation of the information in clinical practice and evaluation. These elements are set out in Table 5.5.

The following organisations (as discussed in Chapter 1) are key features of the NHS Reforms for the new NHS as outlined in the 1997 White Paper.

The National Institute For Clinical Excellence

By applying research evidence to clinical practice it might be possible to minimise the use of clinically ineffective procedures and, with appropriate monitoring and evaluation, reduce risk by providing the optimum care. The National Institute for Clinical Excellence, to be established, functions to give coherence

---

Table 5.5 Clinical effectiveness

- The production of evidence through research and scientific review.
- The production and dissemination of evidence-based clinical guidelines.
- The implementation of evidence-based, cost-effective practice through education and change-management.
- The evaluation of compliance to agreed practice guidance and evaluation of patient outcomes including clinical audit.

to information in this area by producing and disseminating clinical guidelines, evidence on clinical and cost effectiveness and advice on clinical audit methodologies.

The primary care groups have a considerable financial and clinical responsibility in purchasing healthcare on behalf of their local populations and they will need to work cooperatively with other organisations and the health authority to negotiate a fair budget, and plan strategically to avoid duplication of expenditure and not destabilise local providers through poor decision making. They may also inherit financial deficits built up by predecessor fund-holders and will need clear agreements on how to spread the risk and how, if applicable, to use savings yielded through prudent use of their budgets for healthcare. All this will have clinical risk implications.

The primary care groups will be responsible for ensuring that the healthcare they purchase is of high quality. This will be through the establishment of clinical governance for trusts and will need to be reinforced through the service level agreements between the primary care groups and providers. As part of this process, GPs, as clinicians, are well placed to negotiate clinical guidelines for care and other clinical quality issues.

The Commission For Health Improvement

The Commission for Health Improvement, a new body to be established, is to ensure the introduction of clinical governance and so provide support to primary care groups requiring further help in this area.

Access to tertiary care

One of the most problematic clinical and financial decisions concerns who is to have access to tertiary (specialist) medical care, e.g. for a bone marrow transplant, the treatment of haemophilia or interferon for certain types of multiple sclerosis and so on. By their very nature, these conditions are rare and therefore the treatment is expensive. Health authorities (and soon primary care groups will need to) have set up panels of clinical experts who assess the requests for such care (extra contractual referrals – ECRs) based on each individual's clinical need and determine whether the patient can have access to that care. A further risk is the management of such referrals. Currently, each referral is very closely monitored, checked and rechecked through the system which is intensive on administration costs. There is the intention to reduce the administrative costs of managing ECRs which logically could return more resources to direct patient care. However, if the monitoring of the ECRs is not closely audited, there could potentially be abuse of the system as cash-starved providers try to claim more funding than they are entitled to thereby reducing the amount available for other patient care.

Community nursing staff

Community nurses are emerging as new key players in primary care groups. Many new tasks will be required of them including commissioning, negotiation and evaluation skills. With this new responsibility are associated new risks for this clinical profession as they learn to work as full partners with their GP colleagues. As stated by Wilson there is an essential need for nurses to be more involved in the development of PCGs[19]:

Within the White Paper there is a clear role outlined for nursing and the importance of working in partnership. To date there has been no formal involvement of the nursing profession in the management of fundholding, although nurses have been involved at the periphery in some of the locality commissioning initiatives This lack of involvement has resulted in confusion about how to proceed and consternation among nurses, with in particular, feelings of being largely marginalised. Specialist nurses, practice nurses and all community nurses have to get their act together to ensure that they are included in each step of the developments and that they are strongly represented at all structural levels of the PCGs. Many of the concerns being voiced by nurses are the fears of the PCGs being dominated by the general practitioners and that they are not involved in the discussions and feelings of being expected to 'fit in'. There are also worries about the future of community trusts with particular concerns on human resource issues. Will the GPs employ community staff in the future? How can independent contractors employ large groups of staff? All healthcare professionals are employed by the NHS using public money which needs to be accounted for but there needs to be a shared governance model with a clear vision for staff to work towards. There are inevitable concerns about the lack of communication across different professional groups and within the same professional group. All primary care staff need to be involved in developments and have a valuable contribution to make. They also need access to training and time allocated to allow them to fully participate. Nurses have to ensure that they are involved and use their professional organisation to work with them on developing their roles and responsibilities. The constitution of the new groups and issues of membership, representation and mandate will need to be resolved and new and more collaborative ways of working need to be developed. Nurses have to be empowered to allow them to be developed and part of the total process.

OTHER PRIMARY CARE PRACTITIONERS (DENTISTS, PHARMACISTS AND OPTOMETRISTS)

Although these practitioners provide a more 'specialist' type of service, they face similar risks to general medical practitioners in the running of their business and in the clinical arena.

For dentists and optometrists the change in their contracts and service provision initiated in the early 1990s has resulted in a fairly large scale transfer to the private sector as the restriction of NHS-funded care meant that they would be no longer viable as a business if solely dependent on that particular source of income.

In recognition of this situation arising from concerns voiced by the practitioners as well as patients who were denied access to NHS care, the fundamental review of dental remuneration attempted to consider the options for a better system of funding for dental services[20]. This, however, did not produce a consensus on the best method of funding dental services and thus did not herald a move back to the NHS by dentists. There have been some schemes such as the establishment of salaried dentists and emergency dental services but these have been targeted at deprived areas of the country. NHS dental care seems, for the foreseeable future, a great financial risk for the general dental practitioner as there is no similar support for surgery premises or staffing by the NHS as there is for family doctors.

Flexibility in the provision of general dental services, however, has been introduced through the piloting of personal dental services under the NHS (Primary Care) Act 1997. Like the personal medical services, the pilots will be testing a number of areas such as new remuneration arrangements to help target local priorities, new service configurations e.g. better integration of community dental services with general dental services, changes in skill mix, with, for example, greater use of dental therapists alongside dentists and hygienists and more dental services in the community setting, e.g. orthodontists[21].

The risks of providing such new services would be similar to those discussed for GPs above, albeit in a narrower area of care.

In terms of support from the NHS, the community pharmacist receives this via the essential small pharmacy scheme which ensures that people, particularly in rural areas, have access to a chemist for the dispensing of their prescriptions. This allowance ensures that the pharmacist is viable which would not be the case if they were to be dependent on the dispensing of prescriptions alone.

Pharmacists and optometrists have taken the initiative and developed a wider range of clinical services other than those determined by their contract. For example, more pharmacists are providing advice on health promotion and over-the-counter medicines to the general public, oxygen therapy services, services to residential and nursing homes and prescribing advice to GPs[22]. The latter will become increasingly important as primary care groups seek to manage their prescribing budgets better through more effective prescribing, improvement of patient compliance with medication and monitoring of prescription fraud.

Optometrists are becoming involved in developing services for retinopathy screening and the monitoring of glaucoma as part of an integrated system of care.

Some of these initiatives have been dependent on the ability of health authorities to find the funding from their own resources and have therefore developed in a patchy manner. Again, as with the GPs, an increase in the range of clinical services exposes the practitioner to greater clinical risk if not implemented properly.

A separate positive move by the Committee on Safety of Medicines and the Medicines Control Agency is the inclusion of all pharmacists (hospital and community) in the Yellow Card warning scheme to identify suspected drug reactions, particularly of the newer drugs, over-the-counter medicines and unlicensed herbal products from April 1997[23]. The reporting scheme has been launched in four UK regions and could be extended following evaluation. It would not require much of leap of imagination for the specialist nurses to be included, especially as nurse prescribing is to be expanded.

Dentists, pharmacists and optometrists are subject to the same responsibilities as the general practitioners with respect to the standard of clinical care they provide and the making of appropriate referrals to other health services. The new NHS complaints procedure is applicable to these practitioners even if their NHS practice is small. Continuing professional training and education and clinical audit are not compulsory although are considered good practice.

RISKS IN PRIMARY CARE

There is no doubt that primary care presents a multitude of risks to the practitioner who works in this setting and that these risks are constantly changing either by the external environment, such as increased patient demand and changes in the contractual framework and government policy, or internally, through the development of the skills and interests of the individual clinician. This process has been recognised formally and has been facilitated through various policy initiatives which have the function of pushing the frontiers of primary care further and providing greater responsibilities.

The challenge for the health professional and for primary care groups is to take advantage of the benefits of the exciting future presented in primary care fully armed with the strategies to cope with the myriad of potential risks they may encounter along this path.

REFERENCES

1. Department of Health (1989) *Working for Patients*. HMSO: London.
2. Department of Health (1990) *NHS and Community Care Act*. HMSO: London.
3. Department of Health (1989) *Terms of Service for Doctors in General Practice*. HMSO: London.
4. Department of Health (1997) *The New NHS, Modern, Dependable*. Cmnd 3807. HMSO: London.
5. Department of Health (1994) *Developing NHS Purchasing and GP Fundholding*. EL (94) 79, NHS Executive,
6. Department of Health (1998) *The New NHS, Modern and Dependable. Establishing Primary Care Groups*. Health Service Circular 1998/065, NHS Executive: Leeds.
7. Department of Health (1996) *The Statement of Fees and Allowances Payable to General Medical Practitioners in England and Wales*. Department of Health, Welsh Office.

8. Department of Health (1996) *Primary Care: Delivering the Future.* Cmnd 3512. HMSO: London.
9. Department of Health (1996) *Primary Care: The Future; Choice and Opportunity.* Cmnd 3390. HMSO: London.
10. Medical Practices Committee (1996) *Recruitment Survey of England and Wales.* Medical Practices Committee: London.
11. Wilson, J. H. (1996) *Integrated Care Management: The Path to Success.* Butterworth-Heinemann: Oxford.
12. Department of Health (1997) *Personal Medical Services Pilots and the NHS (Primary Care) Act 1997.* EL(97)27, NHS Executive: Leeds.
13. British Medical Association (1996) *Core Services: Taking the Initiative.* BMA: London.
14. Speech by Frank Dobson, Secretary of State for Health, to the Annual Congress of the Royal College of Nursing, 20 April 1998. Press release, Department of Health: London.
15. General Medical Council (1995) *Good Medical Practice: Guidance from the General Medical Council, 1995.* General Medical Council: London.
16. Centre for Health Economics (1997) *Evaluation of Nurse Prescribing: Final Report.* University of York, and Department of Nursing, University of Liverpool.
17. Department of Health (1996) *Complaints: Guidance on Implementation of the NHS Complaints Procedure.* HMSO: London.
18. Department of Health (1998) *Guidance Notes for GP Commissioning Groups.* Health Service Circular 1998/030, NHS Executive: Leeds.
19. Wilson, J. H. (1998) Will primary care groups lead to improvements in healthcare. *British Journal of Nursing,* **7,** (14), 855–9.
20. Bloomfield, K. (1992) *Fundamental Review of Dental Remuneration.* Report of Sir Kenneth Bloomfield KCB, Department of Health, London.
21. Department of Health (1997) *Personal Dental Services Pilots.* FHSL(97)26, NHS Executive, Leeds.
22. The Royal Pharmaceutical Society (1996) *Pharmacy in the New Age.* Royal Pharmaceutical Society: London.
23. Medicines Control Agency (1997) *Current Problems in Pharmacovigilance.* Vol 23. Medicines Control Agency: London.

6 COMPLAINTS: THE PATIENT'S PERSPECTIVE

Bernadette Maughan and Adrian Conduit

INTRODUCTION

The word complaint conjures up all sorts of images in people's minds. The Oxford Dictionary offers an abundance of definitions including one which is somewhat amusing:

. . . emit mournful sound, groan, creak.

In the NHS, we have a statutory responsibility to investigate complaints, groans, moans or creaks – call them what you may.

The Citizens' Charter Complaints Task Force believed that each public service should develop its own definition of a complaint and apply it consistently across all its services[1].

The bottom line might well be that if the person contacting you believes it is a complaint, then that is exactly what it is. This message was put across succinctly by the Local Government Management Board[2]:

. . . If a member of the public has plucked up the courage to complain he or she is unlikely to want to argue about the semantics or definitions. . . . The key is not to be too rigid in the way you define a complaint: this will allow your staff room to manoeuvre.

The Task Force offered a simple working definition which is both apt and non-restrictive:

. . . any expression of dissatisfaction which needs a response.

As shown above, it is sometimes difficult to agree on a definition of what constitutes a complaint. It is possible for a long and stimulating discussion to take place between staff as to whether the issue before them constitutes a complaint by the definition they are using – even if on examination, people within the same organisation may be using different definitions! However, since 1990 the patients have been able to use the *Patient's Charter* as a benchmark for their expectations.

For our purposes we will regard a complaint as notification of failure to deliver a service of an acceptable standard in the eyes of the recipient. Taking this as the starting point it becomes possible to investigate the incident and report to the complainant, even if that report states that there are no issues for the organisation to address. Stonewalling a complainant who feels aggrieved is likely to lead to more of the organisation's resources being expended later. In most cases, the earlier a response to a complaint (real or potential) starts, the greater the chance of a successful resolution. This, in turn, can reduce the potential risk associated with the event.

In any consideration of the issues around complaints it is vital to stress one important aspect. Saying sorry will go a long way towards a positive outcome if everybody realises that a mistake has occurred. The offer of an appropriate apology does not prejudice any future legal action and may help to dispel the perception that the organisation will not be open in dealing with the issue[3].

WHY PEOPLE COMPLAIN

The number of complaints received in the NHS is rising. In 11 years since 1985, the figures for Hospital and Community Health Services complaints rose from 28 990 in 1985 to 92 979 in 1996/97[4].

A rise in complaints does not necessarily indicate a deterioration in the quality of service, but can result from other factors such as rising expectations.

So why do people complain? They do so for many different reasons. In a study undertaken in the North West Thames Region in 1993, all complainants reported a combination of reasons for their written complaints[5]:

- 90 per cent wanted to prevent a similar incident, to avoid others having to go through a similar experience;
- 80 per cent wanted staff to be aware of what had happened and the effect it had on the patient;
- 74 per cent wanted to obtain an explanation, wanting more information about their condition or treatment;
- 49 per cent wanted an apology;
- 37 per cent wanted staff involved to be disciplined;
- 25 per cent wanted to obtain further clinical treatment; and
- only 9 per cent wanted compensation.

The study further highlighted that for many patients and relatives the complaints process compounded their dissatisfaction or anxiety. Only 1 per cent indicated that the response was very good or satisfactory, with no criticisms.

In essence, people complain because they simply feel that something is wrong. They want to be heard, they want an apology and they want to understand what happened and why. They also want action to be taken to ensure that what happened will not happen again to anyone else.

From a patient's point of view, there are often real perceived obstacles to overcome even before the complaint is made. Many people fear that there may be repercussions from health professionals as a result of the complaint.

Fear of being removed from a GP's list and fear of being perceived as being awkward and that this will be written down in their health records and used against them can deter people from pursuing their grievance. The fact that the NHS is free at the point of delivery has charitable overtones for many patients who are humbled by a sense of gratitude for their care and treatment and have no desire to rock the boat, especially whilst they're in it! Ill-health can also prevent patients from making their concerns known and many quite simply feel unable to challenge what they believe to be a system which they do not fully understand and the professionals within that system whom they feel do not speak the same language as themselves.

In a study conducted by the Market Opinion and Research Institute (MORI)[6], it was found that many staff were not always willing or able to help people who wished to raise their concerns and that people often felt 'fobbed off'. People reported a lack of response to telephone complaints and that letters of response were brusque and impersonal, the process was slow, people were not informed of what was happening with their complaint and investigations were criticised as being inadequate. These factors, according to Judith Allsop and Linda Mulcahy, serve to increase the anger and frustration of complainants[7].

A survey conducted by Mulcahy and Tritter discovered that people who voiced concerns tended to do so to the person they held to be responsible, namely the doctors and nurses[8]. In the MORI study, the survey found that many NHS users perceived medical staff to be hostile to complaints and to fear recrimination. Allsop and Mulcahy commented that health professionals are commonly perceived to be defensive and to view complaints about clinical care as an attack on their professional judgement and integrity This can result in defensive strategies, including denial or counterattacks[7]. Defensive reactions to complaints only serve to exacerbate rather than resolve them. A well-handled complaint can enhance the reputation of both the organisation and the staff involved. Complaints can also be used constructively to identify users' concerns and predict areas of risk as well as enabling improvements in services to take place.

NHS COMPLAINTS SYSTEM

A sensitive and quick response to complaints lies at the heart of a new complaints system which was introduced into the NHS from 1 April 1996, which aims to satisfy complainants ensuring fairness for staff and complainants at local level. A committee chaired by Professor Alan Wilson, Vice Chancellor of the University of Leeds, was established by the Secretary of State to review NHS complaints procedures and make recommendations for alternative improved procedures for the future. The findings of the Review Committee were published in a report called *Being Heard* in May 1994[9]. Following this the government published its final proposals for NHS complaints handling in *Acting on Complaints*, which highlighted the key objectives of the new complaints procedure as being[10]:

- ease of access for patients and complainants;
- a simplified procedure, with common features for complainants about any services provided as part of the NHS;
- improving quality of service by acting on lessons arising from complaints;
- a more rapid, open, procedure;
- fairness for staff and complainants; and
- a thorough and honest response which has the prime aim of satisfying the concerns of the complainant.

A key purpose of the complaints procedure is not to apportion blame amongst staff, so complaints and disciplinary procedures must be kept separate. It is recognised, however, that some complaints may throw up information about serious matters which indicate a need for disciplinary investigation.

There are three aspects to the complaints procedure:

- local resolution;
- independent review; and
- referral to the Health Service Commissioner.

Local resolution

Trusts, Health Authorities and Family Health Service Practitioners are required to have a 'Local Resolution Process' which lays emphasis on complaints being dealt with quickly and efficiently at source where the complaint arises, wherever possible. The aim is that the process should be fair, flexible and conciliatory. The guidance emphasises that front-line staff should be 'empowered' to deal with problems as they arise, in an informal manner. Where this is not possible, the matter should be referred to the complaints manager (there should be one of these in every NHS organisation) who is responsible for overseeing and managing the handling of complaints.

All complaints, both written and oral, must receive a full and positive response with the aim of satisfying complainants that they have been listened to and offering a full explanation and apology as appropriate. This is undertaken, for example, by the trust's consumer relations officer. All written complaints are responded to in writing by the chief executive, as required by the *Patient's Charter*.

Family health service practitioners are obliged under their terms of service to have in place a practice-based complaints procedure which complies with minimum national criteria. Where a complainant does not wish to complain directly to the practice, the matter can be handled by the local health authority acting in a facilitative role between the two parties.

Independent review

The vast majority of complaints should ideally be successfully resolved under the local resolution stage, however, the matter may well not rest there. Complainants can apply, within 28 days of receiving their response to a complaint handled under the local resolution procedure, for an independent review of their case. A convener is a non-executive member of the trust or the local health authority (if the complaint relates to a health authority or primary care matter) who will screen the complaint in consultation with an independent lay chairman appointed by the regional office. The convenor may decide to take no further action on the case, or refer it back for a further attempt at local resolution, or it may be deemed appropriate to establish an independent review panel to consider the case. Where clinical judgement is an issue, advice must be sought from an independent clinical advisor appointed by region.

If legal or disciplinary proceedings are intended, the matter cannot be dealt with under independent review at the same time. Independent review panels consist of the convenor, a lay chairman (appointed by the region) and for health authority panels, a lay member (appointed by the region) or for trusts, a representative of the purchasing health authority or relevant fundholding practice. If the complaint relates at all to clinical issues the panel will be advised by two independent clinical assessors taken from the regional list.

The panel chairman determines how the panel will conduct its business and the panel members will have access to the patient's clinical records. Reports of the panel and any assessors are sent to the parties for checking, and following receipt of the final report the trust or health authority chief executive will write to the complainant with details of any action to be taken as a result of the complaint.

Whilst there is not yet much experience of this system nationally, there is a growing perception that there is inconsistency between different parts of the country and between different healthcare providers. One large local trust has yet to convene an independent review whilst another of a similar size has passed over 40 cases through for consideration. This inconsistency does not help the credibility of the complaints system from the perspective of the patients, their relatives or the service provider. Some complainants view the independent review as the next logical step in the process of complaining, whereas the provider views a comprehensive response to the formal complaint at the local level as providing the conclusion in most cases. This difference in perception and expectation can lead to difficulties. These need to be overcome by the provision of clear information at the first contact between the complainant and the service provider.

Health Service Commissioner

The complainants can complain to the Health Service Commissioner if they are dissatisfied with the outcome of the general handling of the complaint, however, the local complaints procedures should first have been exhausted before a case can be considered by the Ombudsman. The Ombudsman now has jurisdiction over complaints about Family Health Services and can also consider cases involving the exercise of clinical judgement. The Ombudsman selects cases which illustrate particular failures[11]. (These have also been highlighted in Chapter 3 and 4.) These are reviewed by a Select Committee of the House of Commons. The organisation complained about is required to give an account of how the complaint arose and what steps have been taken to rectify such errors. Such appearances can be quite stressful to both the organisation and the individuals who appear. A comprehensive complaints policy, well implemented, is worth all of the time it takes, if it avoids a visit to the Houses of Parliament!

Performance targets

The national guidance lays down a number of performance targets for the NHS complaints procedure. All complaints should be acknowledged within two working days; investigations under local resolution should be completed within 10 working days in cases dealt with by family health service practitioners, or 20 working days for those dealt with by health authorities and trusts. For cases dealt with under independent review, the target for completing these is within three months for health authorities and six months for trusts.

Alongside these targets the complainant's perception of the process will be that it is very ponderous. Maintaining good contact and keeping the complainant informed will help allay this view.

REVIEW OF THE NEW PROCEDURE BY THE SOCIETY OF COMMUNITY HEALTH COUNCIL STAFF

In its first six-monthly review report of the new complaints procedures, the Society of CHC Staff reported that there was still a great deal of confusion and uncertainty with the new system, both amongst members of the public and also amongst NHS staff assisting complainants and those putting procedures into practice[12]. The report comments on a lack of consistency or guidelines set out or adhered to across the country. It found that the decision whether or not to grant an independent review appeared to be subjective, based more on cost than the nature of the complaint. The report highlighted the fact that very few independent reviews took place during the first six months of the new complaints procedure, with only two or three CHCs having had experience of them per region. Panels were criticised for their lack of consistency. Some panels did not interview the complainants and others did not interview them first to establish the full details of the complaint. Although some CHCs had felt that the review had been well handled, some reported that the complainant perceived 'the process to be a whitewash' particularly because the review was carried out by the trust or health authority. CHCs expressed concern about difficulties in obtaining assessors for review panels. Some assessors had to withdraw from the process because the case did not lie within their area of clinical expertise. The report comments on the lack of training for assessors and their inclusion in final panel decision making, when they should only have been there to offer professional advice.

There was felt to be poor information available to the public about the complaints procedure. Although one of the implicit objectives underpinning the new procedure was to simplify the process, the evidence pointed towards the contrary. Although 'simple' complaints might be dealt with more expediently under the local resolution procedure, more complex matters would not necessarily be resolved any quicker because of the length of time spent arguing over whether or not an independent review could take place. It was considered that more people would become confused and frustrated because of the reluctance of convenors to allow independent reviews to take place. There seemed to be far less concern expressed about the local resolution stage which was applauded as working well, with greater flexibility and imagination and a changed attitude amongst staff towards complaints issues. Grave concern, however, was expressed about the handling of family health services complaints and the fact that nobody was able to monitor these complaints effectively was heralded as being the most worrying aspect of the new procedure. There was general fear that GP complaints were disappearing down a 'black hole'. A number of GPs were unsure about the complaints process and CHCs found in some cases that inadequate investigations were being carried out.

Many of the concerns outlined in the CHC's report are echoed in a publication by the National Consumer Council entitled *NHS Complaints Procedures: The First Year* published in September 1997[13]. This report draws on the views of a range of people involved in implementing and using the NHS complaints procedures. It raises issues which are reflected in the Health Service Commissioner's annual report of complaints for 1996/7[14] and a survey of complainants carried out by the Consumers' Association[13].

On a positive note, the National Consumer Council reports that many people perceive that the new procedures are generating a greater willingness on the part of managers and professionals to value complaints, encouraging improved communication between staff and patients. Staff in trusts were noted to be trying harder to sort complaints out with complainants being offered meetings with staff. However, difficulties were considered to be more likely to happen in family practices because of the more personal relationship between practitioners and patients. As explained earlier, patients do often feel afraid to complain about their GP for fear of being removed from a GP's list. It is pleasing to note, however, that this course of action is not condoned by the General Medical Council who discourage GPs from removing patients simply because of a complaint.

The Health Service Commissioner, Michael Buckley, received approximately 400 complaints during 1996/7. (See also Chapters 3 and 4.) The vast majority of these cases were about refusals to set up independent review panels. Approximately 2450 requests for independent reviews were made in 1996/97, during which time 360 panels had been held or were being set up. The Commissioner investigated 46 cases of which only 21 were completed by the end of the year. Convenors are criticised by the Commissioner for failing to follow national guidance on how they should operate. In the early stages of the new procedure, some convenors were found to have failed to seek appropriate clinical advice or to consult an independent chairman, or have gone beyond their role by investigating cases to see if there were grounds for a panel investigation.

COMMUNITY HEALTH COUNCILS, PATIENTS' REPRESENTATIVES AND LAY CONCILIATORS

Community Health Council (CHC) staff continue to have an important role in assisting complainants through the NHS complaints procedure. CHCs may act in an 'enabling' role by providing people with the information and support they require to put forward a complaint. Alternatively, depending on the complainant's wishes and needs, CHCs may act as patients' advocates by actually pursuing the complaint on behalf of the patient. Users of health services are not all confident and articulate and may not feel able to make a complaint without some support. In the area of primary care complaints, the role of the lay conciliator has developed as an invaluable aid in the handling of difficult complaints. Lay conciliators are usually independent of the service and are able to mediate between the parties in a conciliatory and impartial manner. The role of the conciliator is impartial and this has essentially been a key factor in the success of this approach to complaints handling. The conciliator will discuss the complaint with both parties involved and help them to resolve the complaint. Conciliation has been used in primary care for some years as part of the 'informal' complaints procedure in operation within family health services authorities. Health authorities are now required to provide conciliation services for primary care complaints and some trusts are beginning to show an interest in this approach to dealing with complaints under local resolution in the hospital and community health settings.

Patients' representatives

Contributing factors to the success of the response are method and speed. One way of facilitating this response is by the use of staff employed by the organisation whose role is to act as a buffer between the complainant and the organisation. Whilst clearly employees, it is possible for them to present themselves at an early stage in a developing situation between staff and the public whilst all parties are still on the premises, adopting a pseudo-advocate role which can potentially relieve stress and allow a more measured assessment of the situation. Also they can be brought into play when the complaint is still at a verbal stage, the patient's representative acting as a collector of information for the complainant with the aim of providing a sufficiently informed response to remove the need for a formal written complaint.

In both of these situations the actions of the patient's representative can reduce the potential risk to the organisation from a developing situation. They provide a human contact capable of removing conflict from a developing situation and, by rapidly assimilating information from different parts of the organisation, give a complainant a coherent answer which it may not be possible for a more isolated department-based staff member to provide. This delivery of a comprehensive response can remove one of the major concerns with complaints, that of the incomplete answer and the feeling that the organisation is covering up or holding back information. By providing such a facility an organisation is making a significant statement about the way it wishes to deal with its users, whilst at the same time ensuring a close eye is kept on potential areas of exposure to risk.

What is of great importance in this role is the collation and analysis of the activity of the patients' representative. It should be possible to detect if patterns exist which identify that different problems crop up in one department or whether many departments are suffering from similar problems. At a simplistic level it is possible to grid the nature of the problem on the X axis and the area or department concerned on the Y axis. A vertical line indicates a specific issue which is a problem to many, a horizontal line a department with multiple problems as shown in Table 6.1.

An issue often raised by patients when a service fails to meet expectations is that others should not suffer in the same way.

To respond to this confidently it is vital to have systems in place which ensure that where practices require change, those changes are implemented and an individual takes responsibility for them. In the system being described, the analysis of complaint issues, both written and verbal, is reviewed by a committee. The make up of this committee is representative of the structure of the organisation which runs aligned to the clinical directorate model. It includes two clinical directors, a business manager, a senior nurse manager, a service manager, the director of operations/chief nurse and the consumer relations team. It is chaired by a non-executive director bringing both trust board perspective and authority.

The group looks at the analysis of complaints. Where remedial action is required, the group identifies the area concerned and documents the need for action. This includes the completion by the responsible manager of a form detailing the changes made and the individual responsible for ongoing monitoring.

From the fictitious example in Table 6.1, the analysis would indicate that communications were a major issue (horizontal line) and that trauma and orthopaedics seemed to be having problems over a number of areas (vertical line).

Table 6.1 Hypothetical table of data monitoring the activity of the Patients' Representative

	A&E	Anaesthetics	Dermatology	ENT	General medicine	General surgery	Trauma and orthopaedics	Total
Medical care	2	1			2	1	2	8
Nursing care	1		1		2	1	2	7
Other care	1							1
Manner and attitude	2		1		1	2	3	9
Communication problems	5		4	1	3	2	5	20
Waiting times	2		1	1	1	2	4	11
Cancellations						3	2	5
Administrative errors							1	1
Environment	1							1
Car parking								
Other	1		1		2	2	1	7
Total	15	1	8	2	11	13	20	70

It is now possible to assure complainants that where an error has been identified an apology can be made and an assurance given that a recurrence is unlikely.

COMMUNICATIONS

As discussed in Chapter 3, one of the biggest areas of risk exposure is poor communication. The analysis of complaints identifies that most cases contain an element of a failure in communication. It follows that if communication can be improved then the level of complaints might fall. But how do you communicate well? As in one of the definitions of a complaint at the beginning of the chapter, the perceptions of the user are the ones we are aiming to satisfy, therefore our communications (whether written or spoken) need to be aimed carefully at our audience. It is likely that the first contact between the hospital and the patient will be a letter offering an outpatient appointment. This letter must be clear and give the information that the hospital intended. It is useful to have the opinion of an outside individual regarding the acceptability of the content. This has an effect on NHS resources as huge numbers of letters are sent each year; if a proportion of these are not achieving their aim then they have been wasted. It is possible to audit the content of letters to check their effectiveness.

Once the patient comes into personal contact with the organisation then a number of situations will arise:

- Orientation – can patients find their way easily?
- Greeting – do the patients feel welcomed by the organisation?
- Professionalism – are they treated with dignity?
- Communication – is what is said to them understood?

It is not always understood by staff, that when patients come to a hospital it is seen by most as an alien environment. This may cause patients to feel uncomfortable or to feel less in control of the situation than is normal for them. This makes it very important to be sure that anything that could cause confusion or misunderstanding is removed. The use of previous patients' feedback is a useful way of obtaining information on how well services have been received and on occasions has suggested improvements.

CONSENT

Consent is required for all treatment or investigation which requires physical contact with the patient. Failure to obtain consent, which must be freely given, can lead to the treatment being declared unlawful and lead to civil and/or criminal liability. (This will be discussed in more detail in Chapters 8 and 9.) During the process of obtaining consent the practitioner must explain the nature of the procedure and the possible complications, thus allowing patients to make an informed decision. For this to be possible the practitioner must be conversant with the intended procedure and be able to give patients the relevant information in a way that allows them to fully understand and if necessary seek clarification of any points on which they are unclear or need further information. Any failure in this passage of information (see also Chapters 2 and 3) may lead to a difference of expectation between patients and the practitioner, which if any problems occur with treatment, could lead to complaints.

RESEARCH AND DEVELOPMENT, AND CLINICAL AUDIT

To reduce risk and to enhance satisfaction it is vital to be confident that the processes and procedures used by the organisation are the most appropriate for a given situation and that they are being carried out competently. Research and development (R&D) establishes the way that something can be done and establishes the best way of doing it. Clinical audit (CA) monitors how well it is being done and ensures that the standards are being maintained. With the recent challenges to the Bolam test[16], it is important in terms of risk management that organisations concerned with the delivery of healthcare have ongoing audit of its working procedures. Whilst there is a case for the central CA function, it is a responsibility of front line services actively to audit their practice, record their findings and document any changes that are made as a result of the audits, these can then be referred to if a challenge is raised. There is an additional value to the organisation's risk management in that non-standard practices and practitioners can be identified and remedial action taken. From the patient's perspective this can offer a form of 'insurance' that the organisation providing the service follows patterns of good practice which are likely to provide a satisfactory outcome.

   The move over the recent past towards the accreditation of healthcare services may indicate that the 'empowering' of the patient, as outlined in the *Patient's Charter*, could lead to the selection of service providers on their performance on 'league tables'. The King's Fund Organisational Audit Scheme seeks to identify that the organisation uses systems and procedures which are sufficiently well organised that they are likely to produce consistently good outcomes. Linked to clinical audit, which monitors the consistency of repeated procedures, this provides a powerful tool to indicate the standard of service that an individual could expect an organisation to provide.

A COMMON-SENSE APPROACH

Research on complaints supports the view that people want a speedy but sensitive response to their concerns and this is echoed in the wealth of guidance issued on the subject by the NHS Executive and other organisations. It is really all about using common sense and by following this simple checklist you are, in the majority of cases, sure to achieve a successful resolution to a patient's concerns[17]:

- Help the person feel relaxed – smile, introduce yourself and use the person's name.
- Keep calm yourself.
- Offer a calm, private environment in which to discuss the problem.
- Listen carefully and understand the person's perspective – empathise.
- Establish the facts and ensure that you really understand what is being complained about.
- Take time to consider responses – do not offer any explanation until the problem has been looked into but at the same time make sure action is prompt. Do not reply to a letter or make a telephone call in an angry frame of mind.

Responses to complaints should be full and include an apology, where appropriate, and information about what has been done to prevent a recurrence of the incident should be given.

CONCLUSIONS

We have attempted to outline in this chapter some of the key reasons why people complain in the health service and what they expect from the complaints procedure. The revised NHS complaints system introduced from April 1996 was an attempt to address the many problems faced by complainants, through a principled approach, streamlined consistent systems across the NHS and a focus on a swift response at source wherever possible.

When viewing complaints from a patient's perspective one can obtain a very different view of the services that are provided. From an analysis of these views it is possible to make changes which ensure a more acceptable service in the future.

The way in which the complaints themselves are handled forms a crucial contributory factor to the patient's overall perception of the organisation itself – a well-handled complaint can and does go a long way to diffusing the complaint and enhancing the reputation of the organisation. When dealing with the complaint itself, a simple apology, whilst not an admission of liability, can lead to an acceptable resolution. But in the final analysis, prevention is always better than cure – the patient's or carer's view in the design of services can reduce the level of dissatisfaction together with effective risk management measures.

REFERENCES

1. Complaints Task Force (1995) *Final Report*. NHS Executive: Leeds.
2. Local Government Management Board (1992) *Citizens and Local Democracy. Encouraging and Managing Complaints*. LGMB: Luton.
3. Williams, I. (1995) Containing risks in general practice. Chapter 16 in *Clinical Risk Management* (C. Vincent ed.). BMJ Publishing: London.
4. Department of Health (1995–6) *Written complaints by or on behalf of patients*. NHS Executive: Leeds.
5. Bark, R., Vincent, C., Jones, A. and Savory, J. (1994) Clinical complaints: a means to improving the quality of care. *Quality in Health Care*, **3**, 123–32.
6. MORI (1995) *Complaints handling in the public sector*. HMSO: London.
7. Allsop, J. and Mulcahy, L. (1995) Dealing with clinical complaints. Chapter 22 in *Clinical Risk Management* (C. Vincent ed.). BMJ Publishing: London.
8. Mulcahy, L. and Tritter, J. (1994) Hidden depths. *Health Service Journal*, **July**, 24–6.
9. Department of Health (1994) *Being Heard. The Report of a Review Committee on NHS Complaints Procedures*. HMSO: London.
10. Department of Health (1995) *Acting on Complaints: the Government's proposals*. DoH: London.
11. Department of Health (1996) *Report of the Select Committee of the Ombudsman for England*. HMSO: London.
12. Society of CHC Staff (1996) *Are You being Heard? A Six Month Review of the New NHS Complaints Procedures*. Society of CHC Staff: London.
13. Consumer Council (1997) *NHS Complaints Procedures: The First Year*. National Consumer Council: London.
14. Health Service Commissioner (1998) *Health Service Commissioner Report: Investigations Completed April – March 1997*. HMSO: London.
15. Consumers Association Survey (1997) Cause for complaint. *Which?* **September**.
16. Bolam v Friern Hospital Management Committee [1957] 2 ALL ER 118.
17. Department of Health (1996) *Complaints: Listening . . . – Acting . . . – Improving. Guidance Pack for GPs*. NHS Executive: London.

7 COMPLAINTS: THE CARER'S PERSPECTIVE

Pippa Bark

INTRODUCTION

Dealing with a complaint or lawsuit is an inevitable part of a medical career. In the Harvard study, it was estimated from an analysis of 30 000 USA case records that approximately 4 per cent of hospital patients are inadvertently harmed in some way by their care and that 1 per cent of all hospital admissions will result in care that could be regarded as negligent[1]. These figures appear to be conservative in the light of further studies in Australia and the USA[2,3]. Whilst the majority of patients and relatives are unaware of poor care or choose not to complain, the level of complaints and errors indicates that there is a need to improve understanding of why things go wrong in medicine.

So what is a 'clinical complaint'? Typically it is an expression of dissatisfaction with the level of care offered and is a request for a further explanation, apology or investigation[4] by the patient or a representative (usually a female family member). In some instances the complainant may be requesting clinical treatment for the patient or disciplinary action against a member of staff. The overriding reason for complaints is so that no-one has to experience the same situation again and the reason the person is contacting the hospital is to raise awareness of what happened (see Figure 7.1 Reasons for complaining).

It would be a mistake to assume that major cases go to litigation and that complaints are about minor incidents. For a patient or relatives to get to the point of complaining, they may have experienced a series of incidents that have eroded their faith in the care offered. In a study of clinical complaints[4], the complainants described the effects the treatment had on the patient as serious: half reported a need for additional treatment, 40 per cent said that the patient's condition had deteriorated as a result of treatment and a third stated that side effects had been experienced. In this sample, 5 per cent of the complaints were made by bereaved relatives.

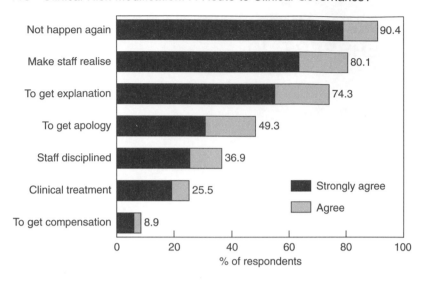

Figure 7.1   Reasons for complaining.

Case study

A boy presented at casualty with a swollen elbow. He was seen quickly, a fracture was diagnosed and a half-cast was put on his arm. His mother reported that he was treated well. He was discharged. However, three days later he awoke in severe pain and was taken back to casualty where he was immediately seen. He was re-examined by four different professionals each coming in separately and apparently not having liaised with their colleagues. On each occasion the examination caused him severe pain to the point where he was sobbing. He was left for several hours unattended and without pain relief. The X-rays had to be re-done twice, once because they had been lost, the second time because the cast should have been removed first. After a six hour delay, a paediatrician diagnosed that the elbow was dislocated and called for an anaesthetist. Unfortunately, the boy had been given a drink and an anaesthetic was not possible until later. The mother felt that an unreasonable delay had occurred and that unnecessary pain had been inflicted on the boy. No apology or explanation was given and she wrote to ask for the matter to be investigated.

At present the number of complaints and lawsuits is increasing and it is vital that a structured and supportive approach to complaints is implemented so that staff and patients can achieve their joint aspiration of good quality care. With limited resources it makes sense to target those specialties that are more likely to experience complaints[4], which tend to be those with high litigation risks[5]. The majority of cases occur in surgery, orthopaedics, accident and emergency, obstetrics and gynaecology, and anaesthetics. In a study of 1011 senior clinicians in the North Thames region, approximately 33 per cent of

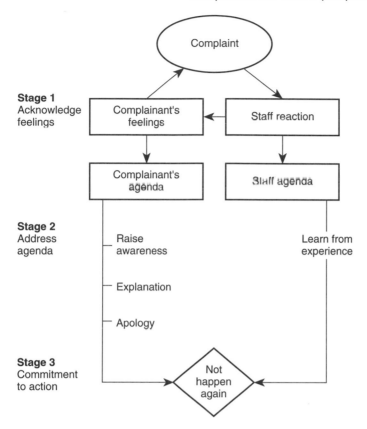

Figure 7.2   Effective handling of complaints.

senior hospital doctors reported having been involved in litigation at least once[5]. The figure was higher for surgeons, of whom 50 per cent had been involved in litigation at some point during their career; this included obstetricians and orthopaedic surgeons of whom over 75 per cent had been involved in litigation.

This chapter examines the classic stages of complaints handling and considers what additional steps need to be included so that staff are in a position to satisfy the complainant. Ideas on effective complaints handling have been consistent over the years, and deceptively simple. If complaints handling were merely a matter of offering an apology and explanation, much time would be saved. In reality, the distress experienced by the patients, relatives[4] and staff[5,6] involved is usually less easy to rectify. The blocks to effective progress need to be understood so that ways of overcoming them can be implemented. Training, support and methods of learning from the situation will be discussed so that by incorporating risk management initiatives the number of complaints will eventually decline.

The Wilson Committee[7] was set up to streamline the complaints process and, from 1 April 1996, the three-stage complaints procedure has been condensed into two in an attempt to increase the speed and efficiency of complaints handling, and to encourage those at the front-line (the doctor, nurse, receptionist) to deal with complaints themselves. At present complaints are dealt with by a nominated complaints manager (who may also be the claims and/or risk manager) and/or the clinical staff involved. In this chapter the term complaints handler will be used to cover whoever is dealing with the complaint.

THREE-STAGE MODEL OF COMPLAINTS HANDLING

As complaints have increased in the health sector, we have been running conferences and training days on complaints in addition to the research programme on complaints[4], litigation[5] and risk management. From the expertise and feedback we get from the people involved in these courses, a three-stage model of complaints handling is evolving. (See Figure 7.2 Effective handling of complaints.)

The first stage is to listen to the complainant's description of the events and to acknowledge how the complainant feels about the situation, the second is to establish what the complainant is hoping for in complaining (the agenda) and the third is a joint commitment of action between the complainant and the complaints handler in how the situation can most usefully be taken forward. This development has been advantageous in that previously the first and third stages were largely neglected, so that complainants did not consider their viewpoint had been taken seriously. Acknowledgement of how they feel about the care received enables a rapport to build up between parties and a commitment to act upon agreed criteria from the complaint reassures complainant and complaints handler that their experience and effort has been productive. In many cases it may also contribute to quality and risk management initiatives.

To make the resolution successful, however, the inclusion of the staff perspective is crucial. It is only then that the dual aims of satisfying the individual complainant and addressing the issues that led the situation to occur in the first place can be achieved. Complaints handling should not be adversarial. It is an opportunity for staff and patients to work together to achieve the quality of care they both aspire to. To gain this, staff must be supported and trained so that they are in a position to help patients.

Action to assist staff can include the following:

- Counselling for staff.
- Support from management.
- Support from colleagues.
- Set up support groups.
- Set up a helpline.
- Feedback on the progress of a case (medical or legal).
- Quality legal advice when necessary.
- Identify contributing events that led to an adverse event/complaint.
- Training in effective handling of complaints.
- Training in the litigation process.
- Training in communication skills.

Stage one: acknowledging the feelings behind the complaint

Listening and responding to a complaint is unrealistic if the staff members involved have not had an opportunity to deal with their own reactions. Staff may well find themselves to be defensive, angry or confused on receiving news of a complaint. Unless the staff reaction has been diffused, any response to the complainant is in danger of fuelling the dissatisfaction. Whilst this is more relevant to cases where the person at the frontline is involved (doctor, nurse, receptionist, etc.), complaints managers will also need support on occasions. It is not realistic to go straight from listening to the complaint, to acknowledging the complainant's perspective; the staff members will need to acknowledge their own view point (to themselves or to supportive colleagues). Thus staff who feel angry with patients for complaining ('I saved her life. How dare she complain.') or distressed ('I've been practising for 20 years. I've never had a complaint in my life.') need the opportunity to discuss what is happening to them before meeting the complainant so that the meeting is not confrontational. Unless this is done, there will be resentment at being expected to be empathetic ('I'm a surgeon not a counsellor') and attempts to demonstrate understanding may come across as patronising or disbelieving ('you seem to think your care was not adequate' or 'you appear to be upset'). It is necessary to acknowledge whatever staff reaction may arise before attempting to approach complainants and to deal with their reactions.

Whilst this may seem self-evident, it is surprising how infrequently this is done. Staff experience complaints and litigation[5] as deeply upsetting and many take complaints personally. Those closely concerned in a complaint will be affected in different ways: if they perceive that a medical accident has occurred they may feel guilty, angry at themselves and concerned for the patient. Individual accounts of medical accidents frequently focus on self-recrimination[8,9] with an emphasis on personal failure. Feeling responsible for injuring a patient appears to be one of the main sources of stress for over-worked juniors[10] and many may not feel able to approach their seniors for help or advice. Whether or not a mistake has occurred, staff may react sensitively to any accusation of criticism, and a complaint may trigger a fear of litigation or reawaken reactions to any previous experience of litigation[5,11]. Doctors previously involved in law suits report that the effects were far reaching: half reported that it affected their personal and their work life to some degree. Some experienced strong feelings of guilt, shame and loss of confidence and, worryingly, over 20 per cent of senior clinicians had considered giving up medicine as a result[5]. Acknowledging the feelings behind a complaint, therefore, includes acknowledging staff as well as complainant perspectives and providing staff with time and support, particularly if they are still sensitive to past experience.

Stage two: establishing the agenda

The most frequently stated objectives for complaining are to make staff aware of what happened to the patient, for an apology, an explanation or a request for further clinical treatment[4] (see Figure 7.1). Occasionally disciplinary action against a staff member is requested or small compensation claims are sought (for a tooth damaged during anaesthesia, for lost or damaged property or for small compensation claims) however as yet, these tend to be the minority[4]. With increased litigation claims and media attention these type of claims are, however, also increasing.

To take these objectives in order of frequency, the statement that people want staff to be aware of what has happened and the effect it had on the patient notably contrasts with staff views that they can usually guess when a patient or their family is dissatisfied. This mismatch of views is indicative that staff do not yet have the confidence to approach patients to attempt to repair the relationship with the patient. As this is usually the key aim of the complaint, staff need managerial support in trying new strategies. One such example of a proactive approach has been offered by Clements who, on noticing at a case review that the clinical care during the delivery of a baby was less than satisfactory, invited the parents to discuss what had happened[12]. After investigation and legal advice the trust were able to offer the family support and costs for their immediate needs in providing for the baby, and were active in maintaining contact. Whilst small ex gratia payments are becoming more common, the most notable feature of this case is that even though potentially the payment could have been substantial, the staff approached the patient first. Legal fees were minimised, considerable time was saved and staff were given an opportunity to make good, itself a supportive act for staff and patients. In the majority of cases, many of which will not merit compensation, the principal of approaching the patient before a formal complaint arises is encouraging. The carer–patient relationship is more likely to be repaired and staff defensiveness lowered.

For those who request an explanation about what has occurred, one of the issues raised is the quality and memorability of explanations. In a study of complainant's experiences, only 41 per cent of complainants remembered being given an explanation at the time of treatment[4]. Of these 34 per cent were not given the opportunity to ask questions, only 45 per cent felt they fully understood what had been said to them and 59 per cent said that the explanation did not deal with the issue that concerned them. This latter point highlights the key to successful handling of complaints: that of listening to what it is that concerns the patient or carer which may be markedly different to what the clinician is concerned about. Accounts typically involve a description of a series of events and may be presented emotively by upset and worried patients or relatives.

When the explanation is perceived as inadequate, the reasons for that must be understood if the complainant is to be satisfied. Patients' recall of medical information is known to be poor and a distressed patient or relative is likely to have problems absorbing information. This may mean that staff need more detailed training in how to convey information meaningfully and that further use of written materials or follow-up contact names need to be employed for patients who have difficulty remembering information. Alternatively, providing explanations when something has gone wrong may be hampered by fear of potential litigation. A clear policy must be agreed between managers and clinical staff that explanations to patients are justifiable on clinical and ethical grounds, even at the risk of litigation ensuing. In practice, as many patients sue partly because they want an explanation[13], litigation itself could be minimised.

Apologies are similarly hampered by fears of litigation. Staff need to be reassured that an apology or explanation is not an admission of liability. The Clinical Negligence Scheme for Trusts (CNST) and the medical defence organisations agree that a genuine open apology is beneficial as long as staff do not attempt to hypothesise on causality or to apportion blame. Unfortunately, blaming individuals is still very much part of medical culture and, in some units, characterises medical accident investigations and audit sessions. In many ways this defeats the ultimate aim of quality medical care as staff, fearful of repercussions, are reluctant to openly report adverse events or to accept that their care was not satisfactory. A clinician who acknowledges an error and would like to practice a policy of openness with the patient needs managerial support.

Any apology offered must be genuine. A placatory apology will be sensed by the complainant and mistrusted. Thus if the complaints handlers do not feel that they can apologise on the content of the complaints, they may find it more realistic to empathise with the distress the complainant is in. Phrases such as 'I am sorry you were disappointed with your care. What can I do now to help you?' can be genuine without agreeing with the allegation itself.

A crucial ingredient in successfully establishing the agenda is in assisting staff with poor communication. About 80 per cent of complaints report that they were concerned about a clinical problem combined with staff insensitivity or poor communication[4]. Leaving members of staff alone to deal with this situation (with the allegation of poor attitude ringing in their ears) is unlikely to be productive. When senior doctors were asked to rate a list of factors that were most likely to contribute to medical mistakes or to litigation being instigated, they reported that communication between staff, communication with patients and poor records were the key components[5]. Ultimately, ongoing training in communication is needed throughout the nursing and medical education process, an aspect of training that is still given low priority, so that many of these misunderstandings in communication can be avoided.

At the same time as addressing the complainant's agenda, staff need to be aware of the issues the case has raised for them. Staff agendas may vary enormously from personal reactions (e.g. wanting to clear their name) to political or clinical issues (e.g. where the staff member may see the complaint as an opportunity to convince a finance director of the need for more resources, etc). Whatever the reason, staff members need to work out their own agenda separately from the complainant so that the issues do not become clouded. Staff need the opportunity to discuss their point of view with supportive peers and to think of how they would like the complaint resolved separate from meeting the complainant's objectives. It is awareness of these issues that will enable members of staff to anticipate possible clashes or points of defensiveness, and to think about ways of offering empathy in a genuine fashion.

Stage three: commitment to action

Commitment to action involves agreeing an action plan with the complainant about what steps both parties are going to take to resolve the complaint and what future action would minimise the risks of the same situation reoccurring. Where possible, if both parties agree to certain actions (contacting a clinician for a second opinion, writing down required details, etc.) the process becomes a joint effort to improve the situation. Clearly these actions then have to be fulfilled and any delays accounted for.

Amassing patient views on care, be it through satisfaction surveys or complaints, is only meaningful if something is done about identified weaknesses. The *Patient's Charter* and Wilson Committee recommendations offer a good opportunity to benefit from patient knowledge. However, we must ensure that information is used sensibly and constructively. Complaints databases needed to be developed so that the core contributing factors can be identified and trends within specialities or within trusts can be acted upon[14]. A general complaints report of frequency and type of complaint rarely gives clinicians sufficient information or impetus to bring about change and this is clearly one area where complaints managers can assist clinicians in a joint bid to use the information constructively.

The reasons behind a course of action must be understood. Where an error has occurred, it is rarely the isolated actions of one person that are responsible but is usually a series of errors by a number of staff that together contribute to a bad outcome in an environment that predisposes to errors: tired, overworked or inadequately trained staff are far more likely to err[14,15].

Minimising the risks of reoccurrence involves training staff to identify core weaknesses in the system rather than blaming the individual who happened to be in the frontline. Considering the case study of the boy who presented at casualty with a swollen elbow, it can be seen that the events identified by the mother are illustrative of weaknesses in the system in terms of organisation and communication[14,15]. Often no staff member has committed an overt error in terms of diagnosis or treatment, the aspects most readily scrutinised on receiving a clinical complaint. It is more likely that an inefficient aspect of the healthcare, such as insufficient communication, led to delays or misunderstandings with other staff or with the patient. Explaining to the family what was happening and why (the process of reaching a diagnosis, the multiple personnel involved, the need not to drink, and so on) would have reduced distress and been considerable more time efficient. Closer teamwork in discussing what each had done would have minimised replication of tasks and may have increased the speed in which the diagnosis was reached. Lost X-rays may indicate a need to reassess storage or retrieval of discharged patient records. If staff agree that any of these factors are typical within the unit and could be improved, structured training in communication and team-building may be required so that staff gain the opportunity to have constructive feedback and to develop their skills. In handling the complaint, the complaints handler needs to be able to explain the key points relevant to the complainant's agenda whilst obtaining the information needed for systems improvement.

TRAINING

Training in complaints needs to be highly practical to be effective. Up until recently, there has been little training in effective complaints handling or in methods of minimising the risk of the doctor–patient relationship breaking down. The Wilson recommendation[7], that everyone who comes in contact with patients should be trained in dealing with complaints, is welcome in the knowledge that for some clinicians the training programs[16] organised over the last few years may have been the first training they have received in complaints handling.

Learning to meet complainants' needs (an apology, explanation, preventative action, and so on) is a highly skilled process and awareness of the issues alone is not sufficient to change performance. In North Thames, we have been running training programmes using actors who simulate angry patients, bereaved relatives or patients who perceive they have been victims of a medical mistake. Using professional facilitators from a communication skills or psychology background to guide feedback, staff have the opportunity to experiment on different approaches to investigating and satisfying complaints, with the rare opportunity to gain feedback on what the 'patient's' reaction and thoughts would be. This approach has been successful in overcoming some of the artificiality of role play and, using the experience of the actors, has enabled clinical and managerial staff to explore what skills are most effective with different personalities. This approach has proved beneficial regardless of the level of experience of the complaints handler.

CONCLUSIONS

Efficacy in handling complaints will only be achieved when complaints are seen as an attempt to obtain better quality of care and where staff are supported in their drive to implement improvements. We must move away from criticism of individuals and start addressing the broader context that staff are working within[14,15]. An examination of the system the individual is working within will produce information that could lead to reparative action[15] which in turn will contribute to improved quality and, hopefully, lessen the impetus to complain on that matter in the future.

A supportive environment is essential before effective accident analysis and prevention can take place and there must be a cultural shift away from blame towards active learning from mistakes and complaints[17]. This is yet to be fully taken on board in practice. The personal support of colleagues is vital, not in closing ranks or covering up, but in acknowledging that errors and complaints do occur irrespective of the expertise and experience of the practitioner. Staff who are concerned about a complaint, whether it proceeds to litigation or not, will not perform efficiently at work[11] nor will they be able to provide the honest, open and sympathetic approach to patients and relatives that is advocated[4] unless they are themselves receiving some measure of support. Staff must have an outlet to deal with their distress when something goes wrong. Friends and colleagues play a large part, however there is also a role for outside professional counselling. In the study discussed earlier[5], clinicians' comments on the psychological effects of being sued were frequent, and, curiously, there were more suggestions of counselling for staff than for patients[5]. We cannot expect staff to provide a quality caring service for their patients if they are left struggling to deal with their own anger or distress alone. It is recommended that support groups and helplines are established within the hospital system, both for information and for sharing experiences constructively. It may help staff to acknowledge the frequency of complaints and medical litigation and thus to put their experience in perspective, whilst using the experience to gain some insight into potential areas for improvement.

The ultimate goal for staff in complaints handling is to diminish risks through safety procedures and improved training so that complaints and medical accidents are reduced to a minimum. By supporting and training staff, we are creating a more realistic basis for staff to support patients.

REFERENCES

1. Hiatt, H. H., Barnes, B. A., Brennan, T. A. *et al*. (1989) A study of medical injury and medical malpractice: an overview. *New England Journal of Medicine*, **321**, 480–484.
2. Wilson, R. McL., Runcian, W. B., Gibberd, R. W. *et al*. (1997) The Quality in Australian Health Care study. *Medical Journal of Australia*, **163**, 458–471.
3. Andrews, L. B., Stocking, C., Krizek, T. *et al*. (1997) An alternative strategy for studying adverse events in medical care. *Lancet*, **349**, 309–313.
4. Bark, P., Vincent, C., Jones, A. *et al*. (1994) Clinical complaints: a means of improving quality of care. *Quality in Health Care*, **3**, 123–132.
5. Bark, P., Vincent, C., Olivieri, L. *et al*. (1997) Impact of litigation on senior clinicians: implications for risk management. *Quality in Health Care*, **6**, 7–13.
6. Ennis, M. and Grudzinkas, J G (1993) The effects of accidents and litigation on doctors. In *Medical Accidents* (C. Vincent, M. Ennis and R. J. Audley, eds). Oxford University Press: Oxford.
7. Department of Health (1994) *Being Heard. The Report of a Review Committee on NHS Complaints Procedures*. HMSO: London.
8. Allott, H. (1994) A grief shared. *British Medical Journal*, **308**, 602.
9. Wu, A. W., Folkman, S., McPhee, S. J. *et al*. (1991) Do house officers learn from their mistakes? *Journal of the American Medical Association*, **265**, 2089–2094.
10. Firth-Cozens, J. (1993) Stress, psychological problems and clinical performance. In *Medical Accidents* (C. Vincent, M. Ennis and R. J. Audley, eds). Oxford University Press: Oxford.
11. Hirst, D. K. (1996) Supporting staff during litigation – managerial aspects. *Clinical Risk*, **2**, (6), 189–194.
12. Clements, R. V. (1994) *Safe Practice in Obstetrics and Gynaecology. A Medico-Legal Handbook*. Churchill-Livingstone: Edinburgh.
13. Vincent, C., Young, M. and Phillips, A. (1994) Why do people sue doctors? A study of patients and relatives taking legal action. *The Lancet*, **343**, 1609–1613.
14. Vincent, C. and Bark, P. (1995) Accident investigation: discovering why things go wrong. In *Clinical Risk Management* (C. Vincent, ed.). BMJ Publishing: London.
15. Reason, J. T. (1995) Understanding adverse events: human factors. In *Clinical Risk Management* (C. Vincent, ed.). BMJ Publishing: London.
16. NHS Executive (1996) *Local Resolution – A Training Resource Pack, Acting on Complaints*. National Training Initiative. NHS Training Division: Leeds.
17. O'Connor, A. M. (1996) The attitude of staff towards clinical risk management. *Clinical Risk*, **2**, 119–122.

8 COMPLAINTS: THE PLAINTIFF'S SOLICITOR'S VIEW

Paul Balen

INTRODUCTION

Doctors are men who prescribe medicine of which they know little to human beings of which they know nothing.

Voltaire (1694–1778)[1]

CRISIS, WHAT CRISIS?

We live in an ever demanding and ever questioning society. Citizens as never before are informed of their rights, whether it be those enshrined in law or set out in citizen's charters. Every day television brings us crises and information right into our living rooms. If something goes wrong, Joe Soap, the citizen, is entitled and encouraged to question what has happened. On occasions this leads to claims against the individual or bodies alleged to have been responsible for what has gone wrong. The professions, like royalty, have been demystified. Also like royalty the professions are under attack. A vet recently faced a bill of £41 000 for causing the death of a dog allegedly as a result of negligence. Apparently one of the biggest growing lines of professional indemnity insurance is for undertakers! Solicitors' insurance premiums have gone through the roof and various professions – solicitors, accountants, architects – are trying to persuade the government to pass laws enabling the traditional unlimited liability of an individual professional practising in partnership to be replaced with some sort of limited responsibility simply to enable the insurance market to provide insurance cover at a reasonable premium.

Such a crisis is claimed also to exist in the medical profession. Sensational headlines such as 'cost of medical errors threatens to cripple NHS' present a somewhat one-sided view of the impact of claims on the NHS[2]. NHS litigation costs are currently estimated for 1997 at something in the region of £200m, and are expected to increase at 20–25 per cent per annum, but they pale into insignificance compared with the total budget of the NHS or even the total cost of management and administration. Indeed, in some recent years the cost to the NHS of legal claims has been less than the cost of redundancy payments. The Health Secretary, Frank Dobson, has fuelled the flames with his comment that 'As far as I am concerned the best place for a lawyer in the NHS is on the operating table, not sliding around causing trouble for other people', reported in *The Times* (30 April, 1998) under the heading 'Ambulance-chasing lawyers accused of milking the NHS'. These headlines tend to obscure the fact that without negligence there would be no damages paid.

Another factor in the public's perception of the medical profession is its club atmosphere. If something goes wrong, the tradition has been to close ranks leading to headlines such as 'medical mafia covers up error'[3]. Although these days the medical profession is encouraged to be open and to apologise and explain if something goes wrong, all too often that guidance is not or cannot be followed. The days of one-to-one attention by the same doctor to the same patient in the NHS have long since gone and all too often if there has been an error, junior staff either seem unaware of what has taken place or appear unversed in how to cope with a distressed patient. Furthermore the medical professional, unlike a lawyer, still owes no professional duty of candour to a patient.

Arguably, therefore, the existence of a specialist independent group of medicolegal lawyers who have the expertise to recover medical records, interpret them and explain what has happened to distressed patients is a vital part of the healthcare service in this country. The revamped complaints system, whilst an undoubted improvement on the old version, suffers by virtue of its concentration inside the medical establishment whereas for most patients satisfaction will only be achieved if an independent view is taken by someone they have appointed to review their case even if at the end of the day the information and advice they receive is that there is no evidence of negligence or no possibility of bringing any claim for compensation.

Indeed on the scale of priorities, compensation, which is all that the law can in fact provide if a claim for negligence is successful, is at the bottom of the shopping list of a dissatisfied patient's requirements. The general experience of specialist medical negligence solicitors is that dissatisfied patients are far more likely to request an explanation, an apology and an assurance that what has happened will not happen to them, their relatives or any other patient in the future in the hope that such a disastrous experience will not have been in vain and that lessons will have been learned. Given a full explanation and if appropriate an apology, many patients will not consider a claim for compensation. Some of course will and in law they may well be entitled to compensation. If there is a claim, then it only makes sense that it should be resolved as quickly and as cost effectively as possible for the benefit of both parties.

FINANCING THE CASE

Having plucked up the courage to pass through the portals of solicitors' offices (which all too often are still considered to be forbidding territory), a dissatisfied client will always initially be concerned, and will require to be informed about, the method of financing his or her desire for an independent investigation by a lawyer into his or her medical mishap. Most specialist solicitors offer an initial interview free of charge. For those patients in receipt of State Benefit, free legal advice is available on what used to be known as the Green Form Scheme, now simply the Legal Advice Scheme. If a claim is considered likely, applications for State funded legal aid can be made. An applicant needs to satisfy two tests. The first is the financial test where in reality only those marginally above the State Benefit line will be entitled and the second in every case is to persuade the Legal Aid Board that there is a case worth investigating. Legal aid, if available, will usually initially only be granted to enable the medical records to be obtained and an independent medical report based on those records. The Legal Aid Board may require a barrister's opinion at that stage, although more frequently specialist medicolegal solicitors are able to provide such advice. Although the Government proposes to abolish legal aid for personal injury cases in 1999 it plans to preserve the right of a patient to obtain legal aid for a medical negligence claim providing they instruct a specialist medical negligence solicitor. Whilst limiting the number of solicitors patients are able to instruct, such a system will at least serve to ensure that, as far as is possible, the patient is represented by a solicitor who is truly a specialist in the medico-legal field.

Clients unable to qualify for legal aid on financial grounds will find that unless they have legal expenses insurance it is likely that the only option open to them is to instruct a solicitor on a private basis or persuade a solicitor initially, or after due assessment of the case eventually, to take on the case on a 'no win no fee' basis.

The conditional fee or 'no win no fee' scheme was introduced in July 1995 largely as a result of the substantial reduction in the availability of legal aid for the majority of the population. It provides a way in which a solicitor and barrister having considered a case can decide that it is sufficiently meritorious to warrant them working on the case on the basis that they will only be paid if the case succeeds. If the case is successful then the English system is that the costs of that case are by and large payable by the losing party. However, in return for accepting the risk of the case the barrister and solicitor will expect a success fee to be paid on top of the costs recovered from the losing party. The success fee is paid by the client out of the damages which have been recovered. The amount of the success fee depends on the agreement between the solicitor and the patient. It should reflect the complexity and difficulty of the case involved. It is calculated on the basis of the actual costs incurred on the case but cannot in any event in law exceed 100 per cent of those costs. The guidance given by the solicitors' professional body, The Law Society, is that any success fee should not exceed 25 per cent of the damages recovered. This effectively means that any patient persuading a solicitor to act on his or her behalf on a 'no win no fee' basis is guaranteed if successful to recover around 75 per cent of his damages. However, the 'no win no fee' scheme only works if in addition the risk of losing and having to pay the hospital or doctor's legal costs is removed. This can be achieved by taking out insurance, the premium for which is currently irrecoverable, win or lose. Nevertheless, the patient has the certainty that the case can be properly investigated and if necessary taken to trial with the only outlay being the insurance premium concerned. One of the unfortunate aspects of the adoption of the 'no win no fee' scheme is that more and more clients have to pay for legal advice out of their damages, when that compensation is assessed already at far too low a level compensation is meant simply to put the patient back into the position he or she would have been had the act of negligence not taken place. This means that, even if a patient is successful in bringing a claim for medical negligence (if the 'no win no fee' scheme is adopted), the patient is less well off than if the act of negligence had not happened. This problem would be solved if the insurance premium and success fee became payable by the losing doctor or hospital.

MEDICAL RECORDS AND EXPERTS

Having accepted instructions the solicitor's first job will be to obtain the client's medical records. The Access to Health Records Act passed in 1990, and applying to medical records which have come into existence since November 1991, provides that patients and their representatives can obtain copies of their medical records or view the originals for a maximum administrative fee of £10 together with the cost of photocopying and postage[4]. If treatment has taken place in the last 40 days, then no administrative charge can be made by the hospital or doctor concerned. It should therefore be relatively easy for patients to acquire copies of their own medical records, although too may doctors and hospitals still quibble about charges and often try to levy charges in breach of those specified by the Act. There is an inherent conflict here between the patients' right of access to their records and the hospitals' desire not to make a financial loss on this service now that they are treated as profit centres.

Once obtained the medical records will usually be examined by the legal representatives and then by an independent expert instructed on the patient's behalf by the solicitor. In the past, doctors have hesitated before becoming involved in medicolegal work but these days there is a greater appreciation that criticism of colleagues or of systems within the NHS environment is part of the responsibility of informed and enlightened medical staff and overall is likely to lead to improvement in the quality of healthcare generally.

Specialist medicolegal solicitors therefore usually have no difficulty in obtaining the assistance of doctors to provide the necessary reports. The doctor used must be of an equivalent status and, if negligence is in issue, must have practised at the time the act of negligence is alleged to have taken place. Other doctors may be required to consider the medical records and to examine the patient and provide reports on the patient's medical condition and its actual cause and to consider that patient's current condition and prognosis.

THE LAW

To bring a claim for compensation successfully, it is necessary for a patient to prove negligence and that that negligence made a difference to their condition. The latter test is called causation. A successful claim for compensation can only be made if all the links in the chain are present. It may be that a patient can show that the doctor was negligent but that it made no difference to the outcome. There will be no legal claim in those circumstances, because the patient has suffered no loss. It may be that negligence cannot be established, even though the act of the doctor clearly made a difference to the outcome. Again the patient will not recover compensation because it cannot be proved that any doctor was legally at fault.

NEGLIGENCE

Negligence means a lack of care. In many areas of everyday life the concept of negligence is easy to appreciate. Most people have experience of being drivers or passengers in cars. If there is a car accident, it is usually very easy to make an assessment about which of the drivers was negligent and to what degree. The test for negligence is simple. If one of the drivers was careless in driving it is virtually certain that a claim by a party injured as a result of that carelessness will succeed. In the field of medical law, however, doctors are accorded a special place. In 1957 in an historic direction to a jury[5] (unlike today, in those days juries were responsible for deciding most civil actions) a judge said:

> In the case of a medical man, negligence means failure to act in accordance with the standards of reasonably competent medical men at the time . . . the real question you have to make up your minds about . . . is whether the defendants, in acting in the way they did, were acting in accordance with a practice of competent respective professional opinion. . . . In the realm of diagnosis and treatment there is ample scope for genuine difference of opinion and one man clearly is not negligent merely because his conclusion differs from that of other professional men, nor because he has displayed less skill or knowledge than others would have shown. The true test for establishing negligence in diagnosis or treatment on the part of the doctor is whether he has been proved to be guilty of such failure as no doctor of ordinary skill would be guilty of if acting with ordinary care. . . . He is not guilty of negligence if he has acted in accordance with a practice accepted as proper by a responsible body of medical men skilled in that particular art. . . . Putting it the other way round, a man is not negligent, if he is acting in accordance with such a practice, merely because there is a body of opinion who would take a contrary view.

This test, if taken as it has generally been understood, means that the medical profession is able to set its own standards to which the court will defer.

It means, in essence, that a dissatisfied patient, to succeed in a claim for negligence against a medical man, faces a challenge not unlike Colin Jackson would have done in the Olympic Games 110 m hurdle race if, when he came to the first hurdle, it was the height of a pole vault.

This test has been substantially criticised over the years but has held up since 1957 and undoubtedly remains the law. It has, however, run into more frequent criticism in modern times and courts in other jurisdictions similar to the British one have increasingly questioned its validity. Even in this country, some judges have decided that they can intervene in circumstances where they assess that a practice which some doctors are following is so unreasonable that they will not countenance such a practice being maintained or at least approved of by the court. Indeed, on many occasions the medical profession itself refuses to defend practices which, whilst carried out by otherwise competent practitioners, may be regarded as outdated or unreasonable, even if such practice would strictly satisfy the so-called Bolam defence. A recent decision has illustrated that the courts may now demand that any practice defended must at least be capable of logical justification[6]. The courts, it appears, are edging towards a more interventionist approach.

The issue of negligence is resolved by obtaining independent expert evidence and it is only if that evidence is in dispute that the issue will arise in court. Then the judges have to decide whether or not they are prepared to intervene and set their own standards or leave it to the medical profession, in which case almost certainly at that stage the plaintiff's case will fail.

CAUSATION

More often than not, however, the true issue in the majority of medicolegal claims is one of causation. The test for causation requires the patient to demonstrate, on a balance of probabilities, whether the identified act of negligence caused or materially contributed to the patient's suffering. The classic illustration of this test was the case of Wilsher[7]. Baby Wilsher was born prematurely. He required amongst other things the provision of oxygen. A junior doctor placed a catheter which monitored the oxygen in the blood supply in a vein rather than an artery. It was checked by a more senior doctor, a registrar, who made the same error. As a result, a faulty reading of the amount of oxygen in his body was given and baby Wilsher received an excess amount. Negligence was proved. At issue remained the question of causation. Baby Wilsher suffered from blindness, retrolental fibroplasia. One of the causes of retrolental fibroplasia is known to be the supply of an excess of oxygen. The act of negligence in placing the catheter wrongly led of course to the supply of an excess of oxygen. The judge decided that once a plaintiff demonstrated that he was suffering from a condition which was a recognised cause of the consequences of the act of negligence, he could establish that the condition, in this case blindness, was caused by the act of negligence. The case went on appeal. Eventually the House of Lords ruled that the burden of proof as in all civil cases, remained on the plaintiff. The plaintiff had to show that the retrolental fibroplasia in his case had been caused by the excess of oxygen and not one of the other competing causes of that condition.

Another example of this in action can be seen from one of my own cases. I acted for a professional man who had major spinal surgery. He was well briefed as to the potential risks of that surgery and the operation seemed to have gone reasonably well. Certainly no act of negligence was alleged at that time. He was nursed in intensive care during the night after the operation and on call was the senior registrar who had assisted at the operation itself. In the middle of the night the client became aware of severe pain in his leg followed by increasing numbness. He alerted the intensive care nurses who realised that something was amiss. They telephoned the registrar who refused to attend, claiming that such a consequence could be expected from the extensive surgery that the patient had so recently undergone.

By the time the day staff came on duty the plaintiff had lost all sensation apart from minor pinprick sensation in the toes of one of his feet. The staff realised what was wrong and telephoned the consultant in charge who arrived, organised a myelogram and re-opened the operation site removing a blood clot. Unfortunately the plaintiff remained paraplegic.

The act of negligence alleged was the failure to attend. Eventually, after proceedings were issued, that act of negligence was admitted. Liability, however, was denied. The health authority's case was that earlier intervention would have made no difference. The plaintiff, it said, had suffered mechanical damage during surgery or a stroke on the spinal cord and once that happens paraplegia is inevitable and irreversible. The plaintiff's experts argued that this was not the case but what he had suffered was a gradual build up of blood in the spinal cavity around the operation site which, if it had been removed at an earlier stage, would, on a balance of probabilities have led to a substantial, if not total improvement in his condition. Time was of the essence, the earlier the second operation had taken place, the more likely there would have been a successful conclusion. The case was settled on the first day of trial favourably to the patient.

Logically, the causation test seems perfectly straightforward. However in medical cases this frequently places the plaintiff at disadvantage because medicine is not an exact science and the question which the law demands is not easily answered by doctors. Frequently there are competing causes for the plaintiff's condition, something the patient finds very difficult to understand. Unlike most areas of negligence, if a patient has sought and received treatment, he or she was suffering some problem to start with unless one is dealing with elective cosmetic or family planning surgery. Almost by definition, if the patient is now seeking to bring a claim he or she will now be suffering from some medical condition. Medical experts have to be asked by the plaintiff's lawyers whether the plaintiff's condition is in any way related to the act of negligence alleged. It must be emphasised, however, that the burden placed on patients to prove the link between the act of negligence and their condition is only proof on a balance of probabilities. This means that the court must be 51 per cent sure. This is not the same as the criminal or scientific burden of proof of 'beyond reasonable doubt'. Whereas in criminal cases the court needs to be 99 per cent sure or certain that the crime has been committed, in civil cases the burden required is only 51 per cent. This means that the court can decide that a condition was probably caused by an act of negligence, even where medical experts say using a much higher standard that such a link cannot be proved in scientific terms.

As explained above, being able to prove causation alone will not enable a claim to succeed. Negligence has to be demonstrated as well, in the same way that if negligence is admitted or proved, the causation test still needs to be satisfied. In a famous case the patient received no compensation[8]. The casualty officer who received Mr Barnett failed to examine him and therefore failed to give him proper treatment. Negligence was admitted. The casualty officer should have examined the patient, but his widow received no compensation because the volume of arsenic he had inadvertently drunk meant that, with no known antidote available, even if there had been prompt diagnosis, no action could have been taken which would have changed the outcome.

DAMAGES

Once negligence and causation have been established, the plaintiff will be entitled to compensation. Compensation will be assessed using three elements. The first is what is known as general damages. This is a sum of money that would be designed to provide financial compensation for the pain, suffering and loss of amenity that the plaintiff can prove that he or she has suffered. Awards of general damages are notoriously low in the English courts. The pain suffering and loss of amenity elements of a claim of maximum severity – paraplegia or tetraplegia – will rarely exceed £100 000–130 000.

The rest of the compensation that the plaintiff receives consists of special damages representing out of pocket expenses such as travelling expenses or prescriptions, and loss of earnings and future losses such as loss of earnings, pension loss, expenses and private care costs if appropriate. It is these latter elements that go to make the more substantial claim and therefore as one would expect, a plaintiff with a relatively minor injury who nonetheless reasonably incurs substantial loss of earnings as a result could well achieve a higher award of compensation than a plaintiff with a much more serious injury who nonetheless suffers no loss of earnings and has no expenses both current and future.

One of the elements that has to be valued is the patient's expectation of life because awards of damages are once and for all payments. However, because there is no certainty in the assessment of expectation of life, there is a real risk in some of the more serious cases of the damages running out while the patient is still alive. To counteract this, in recent years a new form of payment of damages known as a structured settlement has evolved which involves the paying party effectively arranging for guaranteed, tax free annuity payments to be made to the plaintiff, usually index linked and increasing in steps but guaranteed to last for the rest of the patient's life. This can be of critical importance, particularly where the patient is severely damaged and requires constant care but has a life expectancy such that the patient could outlive the carers.

CONSENT

In the medicolegal field the one area where there has been an enormous number of cases in recent years is that relating to the consent to treatment. The Patient's Charter issued in 1992 announced that every citizen has rights, one of which is 'to be given a clear explanation of any treatment proposed, including any risks and alternatives, before you decide whether you will agree to treatment'[9]. Unfortunately this is not a right enshrined in English law. The right to information relies on the same Bolam principle that needs to be examined in any claim for negligence. If it is alleged that a patient did not give consent to an operation, what has to be examined is whether the doctor, in failing to mention an appropriate risk, had been acting 'in accordance with a practice accepted as proper by a responsible body of medical opinion, even though other doctors adopt a different practice'.

Because an operation on a patient amounts to an invasion of that patient's body, the patient's express consent is required and this is normally evidenced by a written consent. In cases of emergency and necessity, doctors may operate without obtaining consent.

The amount of information, however, that the medical profession is required to give patients is open to the conflicts highlighted in the difference between the Patient's Charter and the legal obligations placed on doctors under the Bolam principle. In Australia, the courts have firmly decided that[10]:

> . . . it would be illogical to hold that the amount of information to be provided by the medical practitioner can be determined from the prospective of the practitioner alone or, for that matter, of the medical profession.

According to the court, in that case risks had to be mentioned if they were material and the test for materiality was whether:

> . . . if in the circumstances of particular cases, a reasonable person in the patient's position, if warned of the risk, would be likely to attach significance to it or if the medical practitioner is or should reasonably be aware that the particular patient, if warned of the risk, would be likely to attach significance to it.

In that particular case the courts decided that a woman who had been blind in her right eye since a childhood accident should have been told by her doctors that there was a 1 in 14,000 risk of her developing sympathetic blindness in the other eye if she had another operation.

The English law on consent is derived from the case of Sidaway -v- Bethlem Hospital in which a woman who had undergone a back operation sued her doctors, not for negligence in conducting the operation itself, but for failing to inform her that there was a risk of paraplegia after the operation[11]. The court decided that the Bolam test applied. In fact, the judges placed the onus full square upon the patient, so that if the patient asked a positive question, i.e. 'Is there a risk of . . . in this operation?' then the doctor's duty was to give an honest and truthful answer, but that otherwise the medical profession is the ultimate arbiter of what information should or should not be given to a patient, such an obligation only being enhanced if the patient is inquisitive.

More recently English judges have taken a more robust view than this however. For example, in a 1994 case a judge noted that[12]:

> In my judgement by 1988, although some surgeons may still not have been warning patients similar in situation to the plaintiff of the risk of impotence, that omission was neither reasonable nor responsible.

Even if patients establish that the doctor was negligent in failing to explain about the risks of a particular operation, they still need to satisfy the causation test and demonstrate to the court's satisfaction on a balance of probabilities that if told of those risks they would not have proceeded to have the operation[13,14]. In considering that test, of course, neither the patient nor the court is allowed to exercise hindsight. It is usually a difficult question for patients to answer because they know full well what happened and that the risk actually occurred in their case otherwise they would not be bringing the claim. To ask patients to abandon hindsight in those circumstances is thwart with difficulty. However, again in a case of my own recently, a patient, who was subjected to an ossiculoplasty when consenting to a myringoplasty and had been left permanently dizzy and increasingly deaf, was such a convincing witness when he gave evidence, that the judge found without hesitation that he would not have agreed to the operation had he been told of the ossiculoplasty which itself carried an increased risk of things going wrong.

For adults of sound mind, a decision about whether or not to agree to medical treatment is for that adult and for that adult alone. People of sound mind therefore can refuse to have surgery even if their doctors believe it is in their best interests. So for example in one case[15] a Broadmoor Hospital patient was found to be entitled to refuse an operation to amputate his leg even though failure to do so may have lead to his death, whilst in another case the court ruled that doctors could lawfully abstain from providing food or drink for a patient as long as that patient retained the capacity to refuse nutrition or hydration[16].

The court, however, will intervene if a child's health is at risk and may order treatment even in circumstances where the parents refuse it. The primary consideration for the court in those circumstances is what is in the best interests of the child, not the reasonableness of the parents' refusal of consent. The courts, however, have made it clear that to prolong life is not the sole objective and what they are required to do is balance the various factors involved to decide what may or may not be in the child's best interests. Accordingly the courts upheld the decision of parents not to agree to a liver transplant where the success of the operation was problematic and that in any event the child would require the total commitment of its parents to the prolonged medical treatment and subsequent nursing required for the operation to stand any chance of success[17].

NHS patient consent forms have been subject to substantial criticism. The forms are in general far from easy to understand and seldom make it clear which surgeon is to carry out the operation. Whilst some doctors argue that the more information given to patients the greater the increase in the anxiety experienced by that patient, medicolegal experience suggests that more detailed information makes it less likely that patients will feel anxious or dissatisfied at the treatment that they do receive.

PRODUCT LIABILITY

Consumers in the UK who are injured by unsafe products are able to bring claims for compensation under the Consumer Protection Act 1987 which was enacted to meet the requirements of the European Commission's 1985 Product Liability Directive[18,19].

The main purpose of the new legislation was to improve the quality of goods and services and to facilitate the claim for damages for injury by ensuring that injured victims did not have to prove negligence on the part of the manufacturer or supplier. A 'product' can include drugs, operating equipment, appliances and any number of items used by the medical profession in treating patients. If something goes wrong with those products and patients suffer injury, they are automatically entitled to compensation if they can show that the product is defective and they have suffered injury as a result. A product is defective 'if the safety of the product is not such as persons generally are entitled to expect' (Section 3(1)). The definition of a product includes the packaging and information which accompanies it. One example of the Consumer Protection Act at work arose from an arthroscopy operation during the course of which the arthroscopy scissors broke. A part of the scissors was left in the patient's knee and he had to be woken, X-rayed and then subjected to an arthrotomy before the missing part was located and removed. A claim for compensation was made. The hospital was asked for the identity of the supplier of its arthroscopy scissors. Had it not been able to identify the suppliers, the hospital itself would be treated as the supplier for the purposes of the Act. The scissors were examined and shown to have a faulty crystalline structure as a result of a defect in the manufacturing process. The scissors were therefore defective. The defect led to the fracture which led to the client being subjected to an additional operation. A claim for compensation was ultimately settled by the insurers of the suppliers of the scissors and no claim for negligence needed to have been made against the hospital or its staff.

Wider use of the product liability legislation in claims against suppliers of faulty goods in the NHS reduces the number of claims which are directed against doctors and hospitals. However, doctors and hospitals still carry potential liability to pay compensation if the source of the products they use is unknown or if they fundamentally alter the product so that it becomes in essence a different product, at which stage if an adapted prosthesis, for example, fails causing injury to the client, it is the doctor who is likely to be treated as the supplier and not the original manufacturer.

Other recent examples of product liability claims in the medical field have involved ruptured silicone implants, the 3M hip prothesis and faulty heart pacemaker leads. The Consumer Protection Act is a very useful addition to the injured patient's legal armoury.

CONCLUSION

Patients whose outcomes after medical treatment are not satisfactory should be entitled to a quick and efficient explanation of what has gone wrong. The introduction of a duty of candour on behalf of the treating doctors and a professional duty to offer the patient a second opinion or a referral elsewhere if things have gone wrong may nip many complaints in the bud. The rationalisation of the defence funding scheme aims to identify those cases which truly cannot be defended, and to accept responsibility in those cases as quickly as possible. The experience of specialist solicitors working in the field is that the earlier an apology and an explanation is given and the earlier the compensation problem is resolved, the lower is the amount of damages that has to be paid out. The patient's recovery period is likely to be shorter and the overall cost to the NHS lower. Recognition has to be given to meeting the various aims a dissatisfied patient has when complaining and this is often achieved through the independent view a specialist solicitor using independent experts can bring to the case.

REFERENCES

1. Voltaire (1694–1778).
2. *Sunday Telegraph* 15 January 1995.
3. *The Observer* December 1994.
4. Access to Health Records Act, 1990 in force November 1991.

5. Bolam -v- Friern Hospital Management Committee 1957 2 All ER 118.
6. Bolitho -v- City of Hackney Health Authority 1997 4 All ER 771.
7. Wilsher -v- Essex Area Health Authority 1988 1 All ER 871.
8. Barnet -v- Chelsea and Kensington Hospital Management Committee 1968 1All ER 1068.
9. The Patient's Charter 1992, DoH, London.
10. Rogers -v- Whittaker 1993 4 Med LR 79.
11. Sidaway -v- Bethlem Hospital 1985 AC 871.
12. Smith -v- Tunbridge Wells Health Authority 1994 5 Med LR 334.
13. Smith -v- Barking and Havering and Brentwood HA 1994 5 Med LR 285.
14. McAllister -v- Lewisham HA 1994 Med LR 343.
15. RE C 1994 1 All ER 819.
16. Secretary of State for Home Dept -v- Robb 1995 1 All ER 677.
17. RE T (A minor) *The Independent* 29 October 1996.
18. Consumer Protection Act 1987.
19. European Commission's 1985 Product Liability Directive, Directive 85/374 EEC.

9 COMPETENCE IN HEALTHCARE

Cheryl Blundell

INTRODUCTION

This chapter provides an overview of the law as it impacts on the issue of competence from a practical viewpoint. Competence in healthcare can be defined in many ways and it is impossible to consider the issue of competence without reference to the law. Risk management points will also be considered where they overlap with the law or are derived from legal principles. In practice, the issue of (legal) competence in healthcare necessarily focuses on the issue of negligence. In many legal cases, the central issue is one of causation. This chapter is intended (for the most part), to be a quick reference for healthcare practitioners. Therefore causation, which is essentially a legal issue, is not dealt with in any depth. For a full exposition of causation and an academic analysis of negligence, the reader is referred to any of the major texts on medical law, for example Powers and Harris[1].

THE LEGAL TEST OF COMPETENCE: COMPETENCE AND NEGLIGENCE

To establish legal liability, a plaintiff needs to show that a legal duty of care was owed by the healthcare practitioner to the patient, that there was a breach of that duty and that injury was caused by the breach. Both negligence (breach of duty) and causation must be present for there to be liability. The plaintiff does not have to prove his case beyond reasonable doubt, but on a balance of probabilities.

Duty

The duty of care between a healthcare practitioner and patient has been recognised since the early 19th century[2]. The duty applies to anyone holding himself out as skilled in medical matters in the widest sense, so would cover paramedics, practitioners in complementary medicine and the like. It extends not only to medical treatment, but also to medical communications[3].

Breach

At this stage the healthcare practitioners' competency will be considered. The duty of care will be breached if they fall below a standard of practice accepted by a responsible body of medical opinion (the Bolam test[4] as previously discussed in Chapter 6 and 8). It matters neither that the body of opinion is a minority view, nor that there is an alternative view, provided it is responsible. Plaintiffs will not succeed if all they can demonstrate is that one competent body considers the treatment was incorrect, but cannot refute the defendant's expert evidence that there is another competent body which considers it correct[5].

In making the assessment a court will rely on expert evidence as to what is the practice of a responsible body of medical opinion. Like will be compared with like and thus a senior house officer in casualty facing an allegation of a missed fracture will be judged by the standard of a senior house officer in casualty and not the standard of a consultant in casualty or a senior house officer in orthopaedics. In the same way, the state of medical science is taken as that pertaining at the date of the alleged negligence rather than the date of the court hearing.

The court will always be the final judge of what constitutes competence, notwithstanding the evidence that may be given by expert witnesses regarding the appropriate standard. In the case of Bolitho the breach of duty involved a paediatric registrar's failure to attend a child with breathing difficulties or to send a deputy in her place. The defendants accepted that the registrar was negligent.

In reviewing the case law Lord Browne-Wilkinson commented:

> The use of these adjectives – responsible, reasonable and respectable – all show that the court has to be satisfied that the exponents of the body of opinion relied upon can demonstrate that such an opinion has a logical basis. In particular, in cases involving, as they so often do, the weighing of risks against benefits, the judge before accepting a body of opinion as being responsible, reasonable or respectable, will need to be satisfied that, in forming their views, the experts have directed their minds to the question of comparative risks and benefits and have reached a defensible conclusion on the matter.

He acknowledged that situations where the court decides that views genuinely held by competent medical experts are unreasonable will be rare. The balance of risks and benefits was felt by their Lordships to be crucial in medical decision making, echoing the ever increasing focus on risk management in practice[6].

Some academic commentators feel that this case has revised the Bolam test slightly[7]. In practical terms the decision is likely to make little difference. It confirms that doctors will not necessarily escape liability for negligent treatment, just because they are supported by medical experts who are of the view that their treatment was in accordance with sound medical practice.

Care should be taken when using a novel surgical technique. However, it is unlikely that doctors will be considered negligent provided they can show their expertise in the technique and that the method was, for them, an option consistent with accepted clinical practice[8].

Can the hospital itself be liable in negligence? Whilst this is quite rare, the possibility was acknowledged by the Court of Appeal in the Wilsher case[9]. The court said that if a hospital failed to provide doctors of sufficient skill and experience to give certain treatment, the hospital could be liable to the patient if its organisation is at fault. The following example was given. Junior doctors without adequate experience were appointed and given insufficient training to comprehend the significance of a monitor giving misleading/dangerous results.

Negligent treatment can amount to serious professional misconduct. The decision in the McCandless case echoed the Bolam test[10]. Lord Hoffmann interpreted serious professional misconduct as treatment that no practitioner of reasonable skill, exercising reasonable care would have carried out when judged by proper professional standards in the light of objective facts about individual patients.

Causation

The plaintiff must show that the negligence caused injury and loss. This is often the most difficult area in a clinical negligence case[11]. The nature of the plaintiff's condition and past medical history should be considered. Sometimes the patient's health would have deteriorated even if the treatment were competent. This point is well illustrated by a Court of Appeal case involving three night-watchmen who presented to casualty feeling ill after drinking tea. They were vomiting continuously and one of them was so ill he had to lie down. The triage nurse relayed their complaint to the casualty officer who told them to go home and call their own doctors. One of them died a few hours later. It was held that the casualty officer was negligent but there was no liability, due to lack of causation. Death was due to arsenic poisoning for which there was no reasonable prospect of an antidote being delivered[12].

The House of Lords' decision in Bolitho is also important in relation to causation. At its crux was the test applicable to determine causation in the case of a negligent omission. Two-year-old Patrick Bolitho was admitted to hospital suffering from croup. He was experiencing breathing difficulties and one-to-one nursing was instituted. His condition fluctuated over the course of a day. On the first occasion of concern, Patrick was wheezing badly and very white. Sister bleeped the senior paediatric registrar, Dr Horn, who said she would attend as soon as possible. However, Patrick's condition had improved when sister returned, so Dr Horn did not need to attend. Later a second episode occurred and sister telephoned Dr Horn in clinic. The doctor informed her that she had asked the senior house officer, Dr Rodger, to see

Patrick in her place, but the latter said she received no message as her bleeper batteries were flat. Patrick's condition again improved, but about half an hour later, it deteriorated again and he suffered both cardiac and respiratory arrest. This led to severe brain damage and Patrick subsequently died. The defendants accepted that there had been a breach of duty by Dr Horn. The trial judge considered that her breach involved failure to attend Patrick or ensure that a deputy did so. It was accepted by both parties that intubation to provide an airway would have ensured that respiratory failure and cardiac arrest did not occur. This intubation should have been carried out before the final episode of breathing difficulty. Their Lordships upheld the trial judge's approach to causation. If Dr Horn would have intubated Patrick, had she attended him, the action should succeed. If she would not have intubated him, the action could only succeed if her failure to do so was not in accordance with a responsible body of medical opinion (the Bolam test). It was Dr Horn's evidence that she would not have intubated Patrick, even if she attended him when called. The expert witnesses called by the defendant did not consider intubation to be appropriate in this instance. The trial judge had considered this to be a responsible body of medical opinion. Their Lordships did not disagree with the trial judge's approach to causation[6,7].

COMPETENCE AND CONSENT TO TREATMENT

By law, how much information does a doctor have to provide to a patient about the risks of treatment? This is one of the most common questions raised by healthcare practitioners and there is often no easy answer. On the other side of the Atlantic, the situation is more straightforward. The patient should be told of all material risks of the surgery[13]. This is the true doctrine of what has become known as informed consent. There is no such doctrine in English law. However, some recent decisions point to a move towards the more informed approach that exists in other Commonwealth jurisdictions, notably Australia. The amount and nature of the information given will depend amongst others factors on the treatment proposed and individual patient characteristics. Luckily, the law does recognise that the need for some treatments is so crucial that a small risk of even a significant adverse effect can in some circumstances be withheld from patients, if to tell them would frighten them against having the treatment. Inadequate consent can expose a healthcare practitioner or organisation to a civil law claim for damages if an unexpected outcome is not one of the risks mentioned pre-operatively. The old-fashioned claim of trespass to the person is seldom used and the courts are loath to sanction its use as a means of circumventing the law of negligence. In addition, the treating doctor could be prosecuted under the criminal law for assault[14].

The law of consent

As in a claim for damages for negligence, the yardstick by which doctors' actions will be measured is whether they were acting in accordance with a responsible body of medical opinion in providing the patient with the amount of information that was given. If they were so acting, a claim should not succeed.

The leading authority is Sidaway -v- The Royal Bethlehem and Maudsley Hospital, which involved a laminectomy of the fourth cervical vertebra and facetectomy of disc space between fourth and fifth vertebrae. The plaintiff's spinal cord was damaged, although the operation had not been negligently performed. She based her claim on failure to warn of the risk of spinal cord damage. There were two specific risks in the operation: damage to the nerve root and to the spinal cord, which combined was 1–2 per cent, the latter risk alone being less than 1 per cent. The surgeon had mentioned the former but not the latter. The claim failed as there was a responsible body of medical opinion which would have warned the plaintiff in substantially the same terms as the surgeon. However, the Lords anticipated the future and in Lord Bridge's judgement at page 663, he stated[15]:

> I am of the opinion that the judge might in certain circumstances come to the conclusion that disclosure of a particular risk was so obviously necessary to an informed choice on the part of the patient that no reasonably prudent medical man would fail to make it. The kind of case I have in mind would be an operation involving a substantial risk of grave adverse consequences, as for example, the 10 per cent risk of a stroke from the operation which was the subject of the Canadian case of Reibl -v- Hughes. In such a case, in the absence of some cogent clinical reason why the patient should not be informed, a doctor, recognising and respecting his patient's right of decision, could hardly fail to appreciate the necessity for an appropriate warning.

The reasonableness concept reappeared in at least one recent case on consent. Mr Smith's[16] surgeon had failed to explain clearly to him the risk of impotence (0–20 per cent) arising from an operation for rectal prolapse. If it had been explained to him the plaintiff would have refused the operation. After the operation, he suffered from impotence. It was held that the surgeon had a duty to warn of this risk. It seemed at first as if the defence would succeed because some surgeons might not have been warning patients of the risk at this time, i.e. a responsible body of medical opinion, albeit a minority body. However, there was cogent evidence that surgeons at that time when faced with a patient with a similar condition would have warned of impotence. The health authority's argument seems to have been weakened by the surgeon's evidence that he considered he had a duty to warn. The court felt this reflected not only generally accepted proper practice, but also a reasonable and responsible standard of care[16]. In reality, this case contains nothing new. It would be unlikely for a defence to succeed in spite of its main witness acknowledging that he had a duty to follow the opposite school of thought. Moreover, the case confirms that the court will always remain the final arbiter of acceptable practice. In other words, expert evidence is to assist the court, rather than to be followed rigidly.

This sentiment is repeated in the leading Australian case of Rogers -v- Whittaker, which specifically referred to Bolam, with the comment that the former demonstrated the dangers of applying the latter regarding advice and information[17,4]. Mrs Whittaker, almost blind in one eye, consulted Mr Rogers, an ophthalmic surgeon. She asked about possible complications, but did not expressly ask whether sympathetic ophthalmia might occur in the other eye. She did suffer from this condition as a result of the operation. It was held that the surgeon was under a duty to inform the patient of the slight risk which was 1 in 14 000. The operation itself had been properly performed. The Australian Supreme Court felt it was for the court to say what was the appropriate standard of care. It was of paramount importance that people were entitled to make their own decisions regarding their life. Breach of duty of care was not to be decided on the basis of expert medical evidence alone. Evidence of acceptable medical practice was a useful guide for the court. Factors determining whether there was a breach would vary according to whether the case involved diagnosis, treatment or provision of information or advice. In the latter circumstances the duty is likely to be greater. Therefore, doctors must act reasonably as well as in accordance with a responsible body of medical opinion and cannot simply rely on the top authority in their speciality. Although this is an Australian case, it has been echoed in the cases of Smith and Bolitho, and could be seen as a best-practice type of approach to the consent issue[16,6].

Some specific situations

It is important from the outset to distinguish between patients who are competent and those who are not. A competent patient is of sound mind, capable of understanding the nature of the proposed treatment. An incompetent patient is incapable of understanding or unconscious but does not necessarily fall within the Mental Health Act 1983. The former's capacity to understand is assessed in the following way[18]:

- ability to comprehend and retain information about treatment;
- ability to believe information; and
- ability to weigh the information and make a decision.

This test is taken from the case re C which involved a schizophrenic who refused amputation of a gangrenous leg, even though he could have died if the treatment were not given. He was adjudged to be competent, the treatment was not given and he survived.

Adults

The general principle is that every competent patient has the right to decide what should be done with his/her body. A refusal is effective provided that[19]:

- the patient's capacity has not been diminished by illness, medication, false assumptions or misinformation;
- the patient is not being unduly influenced by a third party; and
- the circumstances in which the patient made the decision have not changed.

If there are doubts as to the validity of a refusal of essential treatment in a life-threatening situation, an application should be made to court for a declaration. The guidelines in St George's Healthcare NHS Trust -v- S (No 2) should be followed[48].

Minors

Parental consent is necessary for examination or treatment of a minor under 16 years old unless the child is capable of providing valid consent. The court will make its decision on the basis that the welfare of the child is paramount[20]. Naturally, this involves consideration of what is in the child's best interests and the court will hear evidence on the medical issues and from the parents. Whilst the parents' views have always been taken into consideration, the medical definition of best interests has usually prevailed. However, a 1996 decision involving a liver transplant appeared to give greater prominence to parental wishes[21]. There is a debate as to whether this case heralds a move towards decision making in a broader social context. It has been suggested that the true significance of this case is in the questions it poses about how English law conceptualises the parent–child relationship; deals with conflicts of interest between healthcare practitioners and parents; and exposes the limitations of the court's role in overseeing procedures for treatment decisions in the case of incompetent patients[22].

The child's parents were both healthcare practitioners with experience of working with sick children and the mother had moved to a country where transplant facilities were not available. Her husband was to join the family there, later. A liver became available in the UK, but the mother refused to consent and return home, even though the child was not expected to live beyond the age of two and a half years without the transplant. On the other hand, if it went ahead the prognosis was good. Her decision appears to have been influenced by earlier unsuccessful surgery and her desire to preserve his present peaceful life against the distress and pain of the transplant. The Court of Appeal reversed the High Court's order for the transplant to take place, the latter having been based on the premise that the mother had been acting unreasonably in refusing her consent. The court confirmed the paramountcy of the child's welfare but went on to say that this was dependent upon the mother. The judges doubted whether the issue of reasonableness was relevant in this area. This is a highly unusual and controversial decision. Once again it illustrates that whilst general principles can be drawn from case law to help determine what is a valid consent/refusal, each case turns on its own facts. Here, the court seems to have been particularly influenced by the very close relationship between mother and child.

A recent decision has reconfirmed that the court is the final arbiter of what is in a child's best interests. The child, aged 16 months, was suffering from a fatal disease: spinal muscular atrophy, type 1. She had been in hospital for the previous nine months on intermittent positive pressure ventilation and was seriously disabled. Doctors described her as being in a no-chance situation, defined as one where the child has such severe disease that life-sustaining treatment simply delays death without significant alleviation of suffering. This was the case here and the treating hospital sought a declaration that should the child suffer further respiratory relapse or arrest, they could refrain from reinstituting ventilation. Incidentally, two pieces of independent medical advice obtained by the parents said that further ventilation would not be in the child's best interests. Nevertheless, the parents did not feel able to give their consent to what the treating doctors proposed. The court held that where it was clear from the medical evidence that it was in the best interests of a child suffering from fatal disease not to offer treatment other than palliative care, the court should authorise such treatment, despite the fact that the parents did not consent. A declaration was granted[23].

The validity of a child's consent or refusal needs careful consideration. Section 8 Family Law Reform Act 1969 provided that the consent of a (competent) 16- or 17-year-old is as effective as if they were of full age[24]. Parents cannot override a child's consent, but the court can if in the best interests of the child. The section does not extend to consent to the donation of blood or organs[25].

If a doctor is satisfied that a child under 16 years old has sufficient understanding of the examination or treatment proposed to give a valid consent, it can proceed on that basis. These children are commonly known as Gillick-competent after the House of Lords case of the same name[26]. From a risk management viewpoint it is suggested that the following guidelines might be adopted.

- A full note should be made in the patient's records of the factors taken into consideration when assessing the understanding of the child patient.
- When children are seen alone, efforts should be made to persuade them to inform their parents, save where it is clearly not in their interest to do so.

A parent cannot override a Gillick-competent child's consent, but it can be overridden by the court. This common law right does extend to donation of blood or organs. The latter issue is at the boundary of law and ethics. In Lord Donaldson's view in re W (a minor) it was inconceivable that a doctor should proceed in reliance solely upon the consent of an under-age patient, however Gillick-competent, in the absence of parental consent. Guidance should be sought from the court.

No minor of any age has power, by refusing consent, to override a consent given by someone with parental responsibility or by the court. Nevertheless, the refusal is an important consideration in making clinical judgements and for parents and the court in deciding whether themselves to give consent. Its importance increases with the age and maturity of the minor[25].

To be eligible to give consent, a parent must have parental responsibility under the Children Act 1989. In the case of married parents both have parental responsibility if married at the time of the birth. The responsibility is joint and several, so if one parent is merely unavailable, treatment can proceed in the absence of the other's consent. If there is a conflict between the parents, a specific issues order should be sought under Section 8 of the Children Act 1989.

In the case of unmarried parents the key time is also that of the birth. Consequently, the mother alone has parental responsibility. The father can acquire parental responsibility by court order or a parental responsibility agreement under the Act. If parents refuse consent, a specific issues order should be obtained. The court can override a refusal (by parents or child) and order necessary treatment, if in the best interests of the child.

Jehovah's witnesses

A separate body of case law has built up dealing with patients from this group who refuse the use of blood and/or blood products. Competent adults can validly refuse to consent to the use of blood etc., even though that may lead to their death. Competence should be judged very carefully in these circumstances and if there is any doubt an application should be made to the court.

In the case of children, an application for a specific issues order must be made under Section 8 of the Children Act 1989. The court will usually make an order for treatment with blood and/or blood products if in the best interests of the patient and if there is an imminently life-threatening situation[27].

Permanent vegetative state

The first case to come before the court involved Tony Bland, who was crushed at the Hillsborough Stadium disaster. The House of Lords declared that treatment could be lawfully withheld, although it would lead to his death. The Trust's application was supported by his parents. It was held (*inter alia*) that[28]:

- euthanasia (by a positive step to end life) is unlawful;
- doctors should apply to court for a declaration before withholding medical treatment; and
- such treatment could lawfully be withheld where there was no hope of recovery and the patient would shortly die, provided responsible medical opinion felt that continuing treatment was futile.

In the case of S[29], the Court of Appeal suggested that in some circumstances doctors do not even need to apply to the court. Despite this case, it is recommended that the procedure in Bland should be followed and a declaration obtained, failing which the doctor could be at risk of a police prosecution. In S the facts were somewhat unusual in that it was not a withdrawal of feeding case in the literal sense. The patient's feeding tube had become dislodged and the court was being asked to adjudicate on whether it should be replaced[29].

A helpful *Practice Note* was issued by the Official Solicitor on 26 July 1996, providing guidance on the appropriate way to make an application to the court when withdrawal of feeding and hydration is contemplated[30]. The Official Solicitor always acts as the guardian *ad litem* of the patient.

- In all cases an application to the High Court must be made before withdrawal of artificial feeding and hydration takes place.
- If the patient is an adult, the application should be for a declaration.
- If the patient is a minor, the application should be for leave to withdraw, etc., within wardship proceedings.
- Diagnosis of PVS can not be made until at least 12 months after head injury and at least 6 months after other brain injury. Proof of the institution of rehabilitative measures will be necessary.
- The application should not be made until the condition is permanent.
- The guidance provided by the working group at the Royal College of Physicians was acknowledged, in particular that the diagnosis cannot always be absolute[31].
- If there is a material change in the circumstances before withdrawal any party can make a further application.
- The hearing should be in open court, but subject to the preservation of the anonymity of the patient and family.

The full text of the *Practice Note* should be referred to before making an application. Guidance has been published by the Royal College of Paediatrics and Child Health on the legal, ethical and practical issues surrounding withholding or withdrawal of lifesaving treatment in children. Five particular situations are considered: the brain-dead child; PVS; the no-chance situation; the no-purpose situation; and the unbearable situation. In each and every case, it will be necessary to obtain a declaration from the court. The Ethics Committee of the RCPCH feels it is important to define best practice not only by reference to the minimum legal requirement, but also by reference to the interests of the family and child. They feel that the latter may exceed the minimum standards set by the law[32].

Living wills/advance directives

Competent adults can make their wishes known about future medical treatment (including withdrawal of feeding/hydration) in the event of incompetence, in a living will, also known as an advance directive, advance decision, advance statement, advance consent or advance refusal.

This area of law has recently been considered by the Law Commission. A Consultation Paper was issued on the subject by the Lord Chancellor's Department in December 1997 requesting comments by 31 March 1998, including whether legislation is required[33].

The Law Commission has recommended that the legal position of healthcare practitioners is clarified, where they either withhold treatment when they understand that this would accord with a patient's wishes, or where they proceed with treatment only to find that, unknown to them, the patient did not wish this. Their recommendation is that no person should incur liability in these circumstances.

The Law Commission has also recommended that recourse to the courts should only be available and necessary where a decision is required about the validity or applicability of an advance refusal or a question as to whether or not it had been withdrawn. The Law Commission also recommended that where there was any lack of clarity the existence of the advance refusal should not preclude any treatment to prevent death or serious deterioration of the patient pending a decision by the court.

At the moment advance statements, etc., should not be relied on by a doctor to support withdrawal of feeding and hydration in the absence of a court declaration. However, they will be relevant evidence of a person's wishes in the application to the court[18,28].

The need for caution is highlighted in an article in the *New Law Journal* about Miss G. She suffered severe brain damage in a car crash. Previously she had given an indication to her family that she would not wish to be kept alive in similar circumstances. The family were supportive of the application for court permission to withdraw feeding and hydration. Due to the complexities of the case a neuropsychological assessment of her responses was obtained. The conclusion was that, although very severely brain damaged, Miss G reliably indicated that she wanted to live. The application was abandoned[34].

Incompetent patients

The Law Commission recommendations include introduction of a single piece of legislation to make new provision for people who lack mental capacity[33]. The current rules are set out in this section. They do not apply to treatment for mental disorder, regarding which reference should be made to the Mental Health Act 1983 Part IV. Mental disorder is defined as mental illness, arrested or incomplete development of the mind, psychopathic disorder and any other disorder or disability of the mind[35]. The rules do apply to the treatment of mentally disordered patients for conditions other than their mental disorder. However, a patient suffering from a mental disorder is not always incompetent for these purposes in the court's eyes[18].

In a case involving the sterilisation of a mentally handicapped woman, the House of Lords decided the treatment could be undertaken without consent if the patient was incompetent and it was in the best interest of the patient in an attempt to save life or ensure improvement or prevent deterioration in her physical or mental condition. Best interest was defined in accordance with the Bolam test, i.e. what a responsible body of medical opinion would consider to be the patient's best interest[4,36].

Various practical precautions should be considered when this rule has to be utilised.

- A detailed note should be made in the records as to why the patient is incapable and why the treatment is in his/her best interest. The matter should be discussed with a practitioner of at least equal status to the treating doctor and preferably senior, and that (second) doctor should countersign the entry in the notes.
- Whilst no one can consent on behalf of an adult, it is good practice to consult with relatives before treatment. This, of course, raises issues of confidentiality. However, breach of confidence is not necessarily actionable in damages. The usual remedy is an injunction. It is legally unclear whether damages would be available here.
- Incompetence can be transitory and the patient's capabilities must be judged at the time of treatment (and if necessary reassessed).
- Where a patient is under a general anaesthetic and the surgeon discovers the need to perform some procedure to which there is no specific consent, the surgeon should proceed with caution. In theory, the situation is covered by the above rules. However, this does not obviate the need for a full discussion with the patient beforehand if it is anticipated that there might be a need to carry out some further procedure. There is a lot of scope for argument especially where removal of reproductive organs is involved[37,38]. If possible, the procedure should be delayed until proper consent has been obtained. If treatment is given, it should be the minimum necessary to deal with the situation that has arisen. In addition to a claim for damages, a criminal prosecution can ensue.

A recent case has considered the practicalities which can arise when treating someone who is incapable of consent. A 49-year-old patient with near-end-stage chronic renal failure and high blood pressure, needed four hours of kidney dialysis three or four times a week. He had long-standing mental health problems and abused both alcohol and drugs. The only way his cooperation to the treatment could be secured was for him to be anaesthetised. This was impracticable and carried its own risks. The court granted the hospital's application for a declaration on the basis that since the patient lacked capacity to either consent or refuse treatment which required his cooperation, it was in his best interest and lawful for the treatment not to be imposed as medical opinion felt it was not reasonably practicable to do so[39].

Do not resuscitate (DNR) policies and the mentally impaired
The British Medical Association and the Royal College of Nursing have issued a joint statement, setting out some guidelines on the use of DNR policies, which may be applied if[40]:

- the patient's condition means that cardiopulmonary resuscitation (CPR) is unlikely to be successful;
- CPR is not in accordance with the wishes of the (mentally competent) patient; or
- after successful CPR, the length and quality of the patient's life would be unacceptable to the patient.

The High Court has been asked to consider a DNR policy for a cerebral palsy patient[41]. An order was made upholding the trust's policy plus a declaration that antibiotics could be withheld if he contracted a serious infection. One of the medical witnesses commented that he had never worked with anybody as physically or mentally handicapped. It seems that the case was decided on an objective assessment of quality of life, as the patient was unable to express his wishes and there was no evidence that CPR would have been unsuccessful. In spite of this case, a trust should apply to the Court in any case where a DNR policy is considered appropriate for a mentally impaired person. Each case is likely to turn on its own facts. It is unlikely that this provision will be used save in the most exceptional circumstances.

Can a pregnant woman give a competent consent/refusal?

The Court of Appeal in re F (*in utero*) felt that only legislation could impose control over the mother of an unborn child, even if the treatment would benefit the child[42]. No such legislation exists in this area. Subsequently in re S, the High Court made an order allowing a Caesarean section to be performed on a woman whose refusal was on religious grounds. The decision was justified on the basis that it was in the vital interests of both her and her unborn child[43].

The Royal College of Obstetricians and Gynaecologists produced a Guidance Note on the issue in 1994. They felt court intervention was inappropriate and unlikely to be helpful to overrule an informed and considered refusal, even though the latter might place the lives of both mother and unborn baby at risk[44].

The issue of consent to Caesarean section has been considered by the courts recently in three cases. The court has acknowledged that a competent patient has an absolute right of refusal of treatment and the competency test from re C has been used. In the first case involving Tameside Trust, the judge made an order under s 63 Mental Health Act 1983 on the rather novel basis that this was treatment for the mother's mental disorder, the mother having no capacity as she was a paranoid schizophrenic[45]. In the other two cases, neither woman was found to be mentally incompetent in the psychiatric sense of the word. The Mental Health Act 1983 was not used as the basis for either decision. In both cases the (same) judge felt that the emotional distress and physical pain of labour plus factors peculiar to each case (one woman talked about the inevitability of her own death and the other had some history of mental difficulty and had obtained no antenatal care), meant that they were incompetent within re C. The treatment was in their own physical interests as they would risk their own health if they were not delivered[46,47].

In the case of St George's Healthcare NHS Trust -v- S a single woman sought to register as a new patient at an NHS practice in London on 25 April 1996. She was approximately 36 weeks pregnant but had not sought antenatal care. A diagnosis of pre-eclampsia was made. S was advised that she needed urgent attention, bed rest and admission to hospital for an induced delivery otherwise the health and life of herself and her child were in real danger. She understood the risks but had rejected the advice as she wanted a natural birth. A social worker approved under the Mental Health Act 1983 saw the patient together with two doctors. The advice was repeated and S repeated her refusal. The social worker made an application under Section 2 of the Mental Health Act 1983 for S's admission to Springfield Hospital for assessment. The doctor signed the necessary papers and S was admitted against her will. Later the same day she was transferred to St George's Hospital against her will. In view of her continuing adamant refusal to treatment an application was made *ex parte* on behalf of the Trust at the High Court. The High Court made an order dispensing with S's consent to treatment. The medical procedures were carried out including a Caesarean section which led to the delivery of a baby girl. On 30 April S was returned to Springfield and on 2 May her detention under the Act was terminated. During the period of detention, no specific treatment for mental disorder or mental illness was prescribed[48].

Patients L and MB had needle phobia rather than any psychiatric history. Thus they were unable to consent to a Caesarean section because they were unable to consent to the anaesthetic. In both cases the court held (in MB the Court of Appeal) that the needle phobia was an impairment of the patient's mental function which made her temporarily incompetent. Therefore the doctors were free to administer the anaesthetic if it were in her best interests. It was accepted that both the anaesthetic and the Caesarean section were in the best interests of the patient[49,50].

In re MB the Court of Appeal set out some procedural guidelines, which in turn have been issued by the DOH as guidelines to doctors, nurses and midwives working in the NHS[51].

1. An application for a declaration should only be made if the capacity of the patient (to consent or refuse) is in issue.
2. Doctors should seek a ruling from the court on the issue of competence.
3. Potential problems should be identified as early as possible so that both hospital and patient can seek legal advice.
4. Non-urgent cases should be brought to court as soon as possible. Where possible, the court should be given the opportunity to hear oral evidence.
5. The hearing should be *inter partes*.
6. The mother should be represented, unless she does not wish to be. If she is unconscious, a guardian *ad litem* should be appointed for her.

7. The Official Solicitor should be notified of all applications to court, to act as *amicus curiae*.
8. Psychiatric evidence should be available regarding competence, should that be in issue.
9. The person giving evidence as to capacity should be made aware of the court's observations in re MB.
10. The judge should be provided with information about the circumstances of the patient and any relevant background.

In practical terms it may be difficult to avoid late applications. None of the reported cases involve a mother who made her refusal obvious at the commencement of pregnancy. One woman had received no antenatal care. Best antenatal practice could be to explain what might be necessary in an acute scenario, obtaining the patient's views, explaining the consequences of a refusal and noting all this in the records. If the patient refuses to consent to particular treatment, it may be wise to obtain a second clinical opinion. If the patient remains competent at the time of the treatment, the consent form should cover the fact that the patient understands the consequences of her refusal of treatment.

In May 1998 the Court of Appeal overturned the High Court decision in St George's Healthcare -v- S and confirmed that a competent patient can refuse treatment, even if that refusal may lead to her death and consequently that of her fetus. On 30 July 1998 the Court of Appeal issued some guidelines on consent which apply not only to female patients and Caesarean sections but to patients generally. For the most part these override the guidelines in re MB, subject to the reference at item (5) below.

1. In principal, a patient could remain competent, notwithstanding detention under the Mental Health Act 1983.
2. An application for a declaration to the High Court is pointless if the patient is competent. The patient could refuse consent to treatment and in that situation the advice given to the patient should be recorded. The Court of Appeal commented that for their own protection hospitals should seek unequivocal assurances from the patient, to be recorded in writing that the refusal represented an informed decision. If the patient was unwilling to record something in writing, that should be noted by the hospital in writing in the records as well. These written indications were not disclaimers, merely evidence.
3. Patients incapable of giving or refusing consent, whether permanently or temporarily, should be treated in what is considered to be their best interests. If an advance directive has been given by the patient before incapacity, the treatment and care should normally follow it. Nevertheless if there is a reason to doubt the reliability of the directive then an application for a declaration could be made.
4. The hospital should identify as soon as possible whether there is concern about a patient's competence.

5. If the capacity of the patient is seriously in doubt, it should be assessed as a matter of priority. In some cases a GP or other responsible doctor might be sufficiently qualified to make the assessment, but in other complex cases, the issue should be examined by an independent psychiatrist, ideally one approved under Section 12(2) of the Mental Health Act 1983. If following that assessment there remains a serious doubt about competence, the psychiatrist should further consider whether the patient is incapable by reason of mental disorder of managing his/her property or affairs. If the latter is the case, the patient would require a guardian *ad litem* in any court proceedings and the hospital should seek legal advice as quickly as possible. If a declaration is to be sought the patient's solicitor should be informed immediately and if practicable should have a proper opportunity to take instructions and apply for legal aid where necessary. Potential witnesses for the hospital should be made aware of the criteria laid down in re MB plus the guidance issued by the Department of Health and the British Medical Association.

6. If a patient is unable to instruct solicitors or believed incapable of doing so, the hospital or its legal advisers must notify the Official Solicitor.

7. The hearing before the judge should be *inter partes*. Any order made in the patient's absence would not be binding unless the patient was represented either by a guardian *ad litem* (if incapable of giving instructions) or by counsel or solicitor (if capable of giving instructions). Consequently, a declaration granted *ex parte* is of no assistance to the hospital.

8. The judge should be provided with accurate and relevant information including reasons for the proposed treatment, risks involved in proceeding and not proceeding with it, whether any alternative existed and the reason why the patient is refusing the treatment. The judge will need sufficient information to reach an informed conclusion about the patient's capacity and where it arose, the issue of best interest.

9. In applications for emergency orders from the High Court made without first issuing and serving applications with evidence in support, legal advisers have a duty to comply with the procedural requirements of the court as soon as possible after the urgent hearing.

10. It is acknowledged that there could be occasions when assuming a serious question arose about the competence of the patient, the situation could be so urgent and the consequences so desperate that it was impracticable to attempt to comply with the guidelines. The sort of situation envisaged is where delay itself might cause serious damage to the patient's health or put life at risk.

The bulk of press commentary has been about legal claims for Caesareans that patients did not want. Whilst this might be the most obvious area of potential claim, others should not be overlooked. A claim could arise from negligent assessment of competence exposing the patient to harm from her own refusal.

This hypothesis has been tested in a different medical scenario where a patient who was a known suicide risk successfully sued for injuries sustained when he jumped from a hospital window, whilst unsupervised[52].

The consent form

The form should mention that the nature and effect of the treatment; its major and characteristic risks; and available alternatives and the type of anaesthetic have been explained. The actual risks of any particular treatment will form part of the discussion between doctor and patient. What constitutes the nature and effect and major and characteristic risks is not always clear as there appears to be some overlap in the phraseology. What exactly is intended? It will depend to a great extent on the actual treatment, but a vasectomy operation provides a good illustration of what is meant by the phrases. The nature and effect of the treatment is to render the man incapable of having (more) children and an integral part of this is the irreversible nature of the process. The major and characteristic risk is that pregnancy can ensue in spite of the procedure and thus the need for contraception until there are clear sperm tests is mentioned. Any available alternative to a procedure should be mentioned if both this and the intended procedure achieve the same result but one carries a higher risk than the other. Whilst some of the consequences of a general or local anaesthetic do on occasions need explaining, e.g. inadvisability of driving after the procedure, this provision more often relates to specialist techniques which carry inherent risks.

It seems that the 1:2300 risk of recanalisation after vasectomy should be mentioned specifically[52]. The circumstances in which any warning is given are very important. It must be given at an appropriate time and the doctor must be sure it has been understood. In a case where the warning of failure of a female sterilisation was given immediately after a traumatic Caesarean birth, the court considered that warning to have been inadequate. The couple conceived another child and the health authority were found liable for damages for the costs of the unintended child's upbringing[53].

It should be remembered that merely because a signed consent form exists, a trust will not necessarily escape liability. The discussion about risks and benefits is crucial[6]. The timing of the discussion and the way in which it is recorded are also of vital importance.

The Department of Health has produced a specimen consent form and guidelines for its use[54]. CNST Risk Management Standard 7 states that appropriate information is to be provided to patients on the risks and benefits of the proposed treatment or investigation and the alternatives available, before a signature on a consent form is sought. The standard says that it is unlikely to apply to Ambulance Trusts or to (exclusive) Learning Difficulties Trusts. Five areas for assessment are mentioned[55].

Level 1

- Patient information should be available in the trust showing risks, alternatives and benefits of 10 common elective treatments.
- All consent forms should comply with NHSE guidelines for design and use.

Level 2

- Patient information is available showing the risks, alternatives and benefits of 20 common elective treatments.
- There is a policy/guideline stating that consent for elective procedures is to be obtained by a person capable of performing the procedure.

It is understood that the latter point relates to the discussion with the patient as distinct from completion of the consent form.

Level 3
As for level 2 and

- There is a clear mechanism for patients to obtain additional information.

THE FUTURE

Since their introduction as part of medical audit in 1991, treatment protocols or pathways have become increasingly common[56,57]. These documents go to the heart of the negligence issue and their use, whilst not advocated merely as a useful means of minimising the risk of claims, can be a helpful tool in this area. It should be easier for a healthcare practitioner to rely on practice pursuant to a protocol as evidence of competence. On the other hand it may well be more difficult to defend a case if a protocol exists but is not used or is departed from without good reason[58].

Protocols are likely to be of most assistance in areas where standardisation can be more easily introduced without producing excessive and unacceptable rigidity. In a people business, a completely standardised approach can never work. Nevertheless, in the area of consent to treatment the use of protocols/ checklists can help avoid some of the important risks being overlooked. However, it cannot be emphasised too strongly that each patient must always be seen as an individual.

If there is concern about the defensibility of a case because a protocol has not been followed, this is not always as disastrous as it might seem at first sight. Protocols deal only with the negligence issue. Liability has two distinct elements: negligence and causation. Protocols have nothing to do with the latter area where the real argument in cases often arises.

Table 9.1   Typical progression of a high court action

Writ issued	01.01.98
(within 4 months) Service of Writ	01.05.98
(within 14 days) Acknowledgement of Service	15.05.98
(within 14 days) Defence	29.05.98
(within 14 days) Close of Pleadings	12.06.98
(within 28 days) Summons for Directions	10.07.98
(within 28 days) Lists of Documents	07.08.98
(within 7 days) Inspection of Documents	14.08.98
(within 56 days of Summons for Directions) Case to be set down	04.09.98
(within 3 months of Summons for Directions) Exchange of Witness Statements	10.10.98
(within 3 months of exchange of Witness Statements) Exchange of Experts' Reports on liability	10.01.99
(within 1 month thereafter) Exchange of Experts' Reports on condition and prognosis	10.02.99
(often *c.* 1 year from setting down) Trial, say,	01.09.99

If quantum is in issue there will be further directions regarding the exchange of correspondence from experts on quantum, e.g. care consultants, architects regarding alternative accommodation, loss of earnings etc., plus provision for service of a Schedule setting out the items claimed and the Defendant's Counter Schedule in response. These will typically commence after exchange of evidence on condition and prognosis.

A CIVIL LAW ACTION IN OUTLINE

Claims with a value of £50 000 or above will usually be issued in the High Court. Those with a lesser value should be issued in the County Court.

At the moment, a High Court action will proceed typically as in Table 9.1. Deadlines can be varied by agreement of the parties, but the court is increasing its control over matters and this is likely to increase further under the case management philosophy of the Woolf regime.

Although there is provision for automatic directions and a shorter timetable in the County Court, these are often varied and the case will follow a similar pattern to the High Court. In some instances the title of a particular step may be different, e.g. *Particulars of Claim* rather than *Statement of Claim*.

A major change in the way that litigation is to be handled both by practitioners and by the courts was heralded by Lord Woolf's Review of Civil Justice which culminated in his *Access to Justice* report in July 1996. He suggests that there should be a fast-track for claims up to £10 000 in value and a multitrack for claims in excess of this figure. Streamlined procedures will become the norm with a set protocol for pre-action matters such as disclosure of medical records and letters before action, restrictions on the calling of oral evidence from witnesses of fact and the possibility of a court-appointed and/or jointly instructed expert. All these proposals, if implemented will have a radical effect on the way litigation is conducted. The use of mediation as an alternative to the court process is also being considered[59]. The target implementation date is April 1999.

In September 1997, Sir Peter Middleton's report to the Lord Chancellor, entitled *Review of Civil Justice and Legal Aid*, was published[60]. He endorsed Lord Woolf's ideas, in particular about judicial case management with different tracks being established for different value cases. He also endorsed procedural changes to promote settlement and eliminate unnecessary complexity, including the court's power to appoint a single expert in appropriate cases. A unified set of court rules will underpin the whole system. The use of Alternative Dispute Resolution (ADR) has again been emphasised.

Overhaul of the litigation procedure is only part of the equation if Lord Woolf's objectives of fairness, justice, proportionality of cost and speed of resolution are to be achieved. The pre-litigation stage is crucial and the Middleton report suggests the use of best-practice protocols. The aim of these protocols and the associated court rules is to reduce delay and cost, so they must incorporate effective incentives and penalties. It is acknowledged that these should be proportionate, targeted, timely and foreseeable, i.e. a debarring order might not be appropriate where the party has no control over the default, in those circumstances a financial penalty might be imposed on the solicitor instead.

Consultation papers were published regarding the pre-litigation stages[61,62]. A pre-action protocol designed by the Clinical Disputes Forum (CDF) has been issued by the Lord Chancellor's Department. The CDF is a multi-disciplinary body, formed in 1997, as a result of Lord Woolf's Access to Justice Enquiry. One of the aims of the CDF is to find less adversarial and more cost effective ways of resolving disputes about healthcare and medical treatment. If a claim seems likely, a framework is triggered by the protocol. It is described not as a comprehensive code governing all steps in clinical disputes, but as a code of good practice which parties should follow when litigation might be a possibility. The protocol is divided into a commitments section covering guiding principals which health care providers and patients and their advisers are invited to endorse, and a steps section which includes the recommended sequence of actions to be followed if litigation is a prospect.

Commitments

1. Key staff should be trained to have some knowledge of healthcare law and of complaints procedures and civil litigation practice and procedure. Claims and litigation managers are included in the definition of key staff.
2. Clinical practice should be delivered to commonly accepted standards and monitored through audit and risk management in accordance with the principal of clinical governance.
3. Adverse outcome reporting systems should be set up in all specialties.
4. The results of adverse incidents and complaints should be used positively to improve patient service.
5. Patients should receive clear and comprehensible information in an accessible form about how to raise concerns or complaints.
6. Efficient and effective systems of recording and storing patient records should be established. These should be in accordance with Department of Health guidance i.e. 8 years for an adult patient, but 25 years for essential obstetric and paediatric records[63,64].
7. Patients should be advised of a serious adverse outcome and on request an oral or written explanation should be provided to the patient/representative to gather the information on further steps open to the patient including future treatment options, an apology, changes in procedure which will benefit patients and/or compensation.
8. Patients and their advisers have complementary obligations and should report any concerns and dissatisfaction in a timely fashion. In addition, they should consider the full range of options available after an adverse outcome and when satisfied should inform the health care provider that the matter has been concluded.

Protocol steps

1. Obtaining the health records

   (i)   Requests by patients or their advisers should provide sufficient information to alert the health care provider when an adverse outcome has been serious or had serious consequences and be as specific as possible about the records required.
   (ii) Requests for copies of the records should be made using the Law Society and Department of Health standard form.
   (iii) A copy of the records should be provided within 40 days and for a cost not exceeding the charges permissible under the Access to Health Records Act 1990 (currently a maximum of £10.00 plus photocopying and postage).
   (iv) If records cannot be provided within 40 days, the problem should be explained quickly and information provided about what is being done to resolve it.

    (v)   Healthcare providers should adopt a policy on which cases will be investigated at this stage. It is acknowledged that it is not practicable for all cases to be investigated.

    (vi) If the health care provider fails to provide the records within 40 days, the patient or a representative can then apply to court for an order for pre-action disclosure.

    (vii) If additional health records are required from a third party, in the first instance they should be requested by and through the patient.

2. Letter of claim

    (i)   A template for the recommended contents of the letter is included in the protocol.

    (ii)   If after analysis of the records there appears to be a claim, a formal letter of claim should be sent.

    (iii) The letter of claim should contain a clear summary of the facts and the main allegations of negligence, further describing the patient's injuries and any financial loss incurred.

    (iv) In more complex cases a chronology should be provided.

    (v)   The letter of claim should refer to any relevant documents and if these are not in the potential defendant's possession copies should be provided.

    (vi) Sufficient information must be given to enable the potential defendant to commence the investigations and fix an initial reserve for the claim.

    (vii) Letters of claim are not intended to have the same status as pleadings.

    (viii) Proceedings should not be issued until after three months from the letter of claim, unless there is a limitation problem or the patient's position otherwise needs to be protected by early issue.

    (ix) If the patient or adviser wishes to make an offer to settle this should be made coupled with a medical report detailing injuries and condition and prognosis. A schedule of loss and supporting documentation should also be provided.

3. The response

    (i)   A template for the suggested contents of the letter of response is provided in the protocol.

    (ii)   The letter of claim should be acknowledged within 14 days of receipt and identify who will be dealing with the matter.

    (iii) A reasoned answer should be provided to the letter of claim within three months. For example if the claim is admitted, this should be stated in clear terms. If any part of the claim is admitted that should be made clear and an explanation given as to why other parts of the claim are not admitted. Admissions will be binding. If the patient has made an offer to settle, that offer should be responded to in this letter, preferably with reasons.

(iv) If agreement is reached on liability, the parties should aim to agree a reasonable period for resolving the value of the claim.

4. Experts

No specific suggestions are made about the instruction of experts although it is noted that sharing expert evidence may be appropriate on issues relating to the value of the claim.

5. Alternative dispute resolution

The protocol does not go into any detail about ADR. However it does emphasise that most disputes are resolved by discussion and negotiation and that parties should bear this in mind in the context of face to face meetings being helpful in exploring further treatment for the patient and reaching understandings about what has happened. Various alternative methods of resolving disputes are mentioned including the NHS complaints procedure, mediation, arbitration, determination by an expert and early neutral evaluation by a medical or legal expert.

In relation to medical records, to what extent is the 25 year period for obstetric and paediatric records sufficient in view of the case of Headford? In that case there was a 28 year delay between the plaintiff suffering brain damage as a 10-month-old baby and the issue of the writ for damages. The Court of Appeal held that the claim could proceed if the plaintiff was under a continuing disability[65].

Preparing the healthcare practitioner for litigation

Documentation and record keeping

This section will build upon the issues discussed in Chapter 2 and discuss them further from a legal viewpoint. The importance of good record keeping cannot be over-emphasised. Legally, contemporaneous evidence is always more reliable than evidence gathered at a later stage. It is accepted that notes cannot always be absolutely contemporaneous. After all, the practitioner's first duty is patient care rather than note writing. However, it is inadvisable to write notes up in bulk at the end of a shift. All entries should bear a time as well as a date. In the case of an incompetent patient, the relevant entry should be countersigned by another doctor of at least equal, but preferably senior, standing to the treating doctor.

It is easier and less expensive to gather evidence immediately after an incident than to have to piece together the story after a claim has been notified. The Woolf reforms and the pre-litigation protocols are likely to have an impact here. Written evidence in the form of a contemporaneous record is generally considered to be more weighty than oral evidence. However, at the trial itself, the presence of the witness to give oral evidence is crucial. A written statement can be put in evidence in some circumstances, even though the maker is not at court to be cross-examined by the other party's barrister[66]. A missing witness or document could be fatal to the defence of an otherwise defensible case.

It is equally vital for any hospital to have an adequately resourced records department. This item is also likely to feature in the pre-litigation protocol. Strict time limits can apply for disclosure of many records[67]. Perhaps more significantly, solicitors employed by plaintiffs can always issue court proceedings if records are not disclosed voluntarily and promptly. It is almost inevitable that the defendant hospital will have to pay the cost of this exercise.

A library type system should operate in the department. Notes should only be signed out to a named person who is fully responsible for their return. All notes, X-rays, scans etc. should be kept together.

A signature database can be of great assistance in tracing former staff who may be key witnesses for the defence. It would be ironic to find a superbly made record, but an indecipherable signature. The construction of the database is quite simple. On induction all staff are required to provide a specimen signature alongside their printed name and these are kept either as a written record or scanned into a computer.

Drug allergies are another good example of a problem where a few simple steps can minimise the risk of a disaster. In many cases administration of the offending drug causes no harm. If the patient then dies due to an unrelated factor, the hospital may nevertheless be faced with a difficult explanation and some embarrassment at the subsequent inquest. Traditionally, the place for noting allergies is on the drug chart. In case this is overlooked, a guideline could be devised whereby the person taking the first history attaches a drug allergy sticker to the front of the file.

No consideration of record keeping would be complete without mention of doctor–patient confidentiality. The basic rule is that communications between the two are confidential, so prior authority from the patient is required before any disclosure is made. However, if the patient poses a serious danger to another person the doctor is obliged to use reasonable skill and care to protect the individual from danger[68].

Witness statements

The witness statement is the key factual document in the litigation process. Preliminary statements should be taken by the in-house claims manager as early as possible. A checklist might cover the following items.

● Name, address and occupation of witness.
● Position and qualification.
● Name of patient and condition.
● Treatment or procedure being carried out.
● Names and status of other witnesses.
● Who obtained consent from the patient.
● A factual description of the incident.

The statement should be in numbered paragraphs, in chronological order and in the witness' own words. Facts should be within the maker's own knowledge, although hearsay evidence will now be permitted as a result of changes introduced by the Civil Evidence Act 1995[69]. Nevertheless, the latter type of evidence should be avoided if at all possible as its value is likely to be less than that of direct evidence. Opinion evidence should be avoided. Copies of any documents to which the maker refers should be attached for ease of reference. The statement should be made to the best of the witness' own knowledge and belief and words to that effect inserted at the end of the document[70].

Preparation for court proceedings

Preparation for trial will usually begin with a pre-trial conference with counsel. As for self-preparation, obviously witnesses should read through their statements and notes before the hearing. The contents of the witness statements will govern what oral evidence can be given by the witnesses. Whilst witnesses are usually allowed to depart from the strict contents of the statement if it is merely elaboration of a point, any additional information that they wish to put before the court will need leave from the judge. Thus it is important to have prepared a comprehensive and accurate document. When in the witness box, the witness should remember to answer (only) the question rather than offer extra information or deliver a monologue on the subject in issue.

On a practical level, the answer to a question from the practitioner's barrister is often self-evident from the phrasing of the question. It is the barrister's job to ensure that the questions are put in such a way that all relevant evidence to support a party's case, is given. In cross-examination, the other party's barrister will be seeking to undermine the testimony of the practitioner, so answers should be kept as short as possible whilst conveying all that the witness feels is necessary to explain the point to the judge. It is extremely dangerous to speculate in an answer as it provides scope for the opposing barrister to ask further questions. There are no hard and fast rules. Any doubts or difficulties should be raised at the pre-trial conference or earlier with the practitioner's solicitor.

De-briefing

At the most basic level the de-briefing is a matter of learning from mistakes. Two particular issues are worth considering. Why was the case lost? Why was a case that was lost run to trial rather than settled? In many ways the latter is the more important question. It also shows the danger of an analysis of legal advisers purely on the number of trials they have participated in. Whilst this is a valid consideration, the overall cost of the case is the key issue. Thus the total bill rather than hourly rate charged is the true indicator of value for money.

Choosing and working with expert witnesses

The choice of expert witnesses is an integral part of proving competence in healthcare. It is worth looking at the Bolam test again and what has been said by the House of Lords in Bolitho[4,6]. Doctors are not negligent if they have acted in accordance with a practice accepted as proper by a responsible body of medical opinion. Therefore the expert witness should be someone in the same discipline and at the same level as the treating doctor. Thus negligence should be distinguished from causation. The state of the art expert is useful to deal with the latter. It should be borne in mind that there is no negligence simply because there is an alternative body which would have acted differently.

The expert instructed should be of the same school of thought as the practitioners being defended rather than merely confirming that doctors in general would find their practice to be an acceptable alternative. Such an expert would be cross-examination fodder for the other side. The expert must wholeheartedly support the doctor being defended. This is a quite a different matter to the expert being a defendant or plaintiff man. The opinion should be completely objective, otherwise it is useless for litigation purposes.

It is essential that the expert can report quickly. There is often very little time for the defence to prepare its case. There may be even less time when the Woolf reforms are implemented. The expert should be in current practice or if not, only recently retired. It is essential that the expert was in practice at the time of the incident. For that reason academics and managers may not be ideal expert witnesses. The Woolf reforms are also likely to have an impact on the number of experts in a case and whether they are instructed by one party or jointly or are court appointed.

On a practical note, experts should be paid promptly. Likewise they should be advised promptly of any factors which affect whether and when they may be needed for trial.

CLAIMS HANDLING

How can a potential claim be recognised and what should be done about it? Any good untoward clinical incident reporting system should provide an early warning about potential claims (as discussed as a risk modification tool in Chapter 2). Should all incidents be investigated? If not, by what criteria should they be assessed? Where resources are scarce, it is obviously not possible or cost effective to investigate all potential claims. One possible criterion is all potential claims with a value in excess of a certain figure. It could be argued that all brain-damaged baby cases should be investigated because of their potential long-tail and the associated difficulty of tracing witnesses who have any recollection of the matter.

At the stage where a letter of complaint is received there is an even stronger argument to start full investigations in addition to the requirements of the complaints procedure[71]. At that stage it should be possible to resolve some potential claims by a suitable apology and/or offer of an ex-gratia payment. The potential effect of the recoupment of benefits regulations should be taken into consideration. The £2500 small payments limit has been abolished so that any payment of compensation will potentially trigger repayment of all relevant benefits[72]. Recent guidance from the DSS suggests that goodwill payments defined as being made as redress for incidents which have caused distress or minor injury, are exempt. However, it is made clear that where the complainant subsequently seeks damages because a minor injury proves more serious and is in effect suing for compensation, the Compensation Recovery Unit (CRU) must be notified[73].

At some point in the claims management process it will be apparent whether the claim is, on balance, defensible or not. As soon as the latter is established an offer of settlement (or if proceedings have started a payment into court) should be made. To continue to defend such claims only serves to increase the costs of both sides, which will fall to be paid by the defendant.

A legally aided plaintiff poses special problems. A plaintiff has no real disincentive to allowing the claim to proceed to trial. A defendant will only recover the costs of a successful defence if the plaintiff has either failed to beat a payment into court or if costs of an interlocutory hearing have been awarded in the defendant's favour. In both cases any damages awarded will be reduced by the defendant's costs. Nevertheless, the defendant is clearly at a disadvantage. Even if the plaintiff loses at trial the costs order in its favour will not be enforced without the leave of the court. In practical terms the order is often useless.

In small value cases, especially where the plaintiff is legally aided, it can be worthwhile considering an economic settlement, irrespective of the merits of the case. However, this provision should not be used arbitrarily. In a case that may be the start of a series, it may be worth spending more on legal costs than the value of the claim, just to avoid opening the floodgates.

The plaintiff's financial status would have become less problematic if conditional fees had replaced legal aid for clinical negligence claims. Plaintiffs would purchase insurance to cover the defendant's costs in an unsuccessful action. Thus, a successful defendant could obtain more than a pyrrhic victory in cases where costs recovery would not be possible, if the plaintiff is legally aided. The Consultation Paper, *Access to Justice with Conditional Fees*, makes it clear that the Lord Chancellor has not dismissed replacing legal aid with conditional fees in this area. It seems likely that the idea will be implemented eventually, but not until there has been further consultation and some more cases based on conditional fees have been concluded. In an attempt to prevent public money being wasted on cases that recover nothing or very little, the government proposes that legal aid contracts will only be given to solicitors who have shown sufficient competence in this area, for example by membership of the Law Society Medical Negligence or AVMA panels. Comments on the consultation paper were invited by 30 April 1998[74].

CONCLUSIONS

The legal implications of any step taken regarding potential litigation should always be considered. Sometimes patients or their family will ask for an apology, the implication often being that the matter will not be taken any further if a response satisfactory to the patient is received. From a legal viewpoint there are a number of matters that need to be considered. The timing of an apology is likely to be such that it will not be privileged from disclosure in any future court proceedings. This factor causes much concern. In many ways the concern is unwarranted, but it is important to consider the likely outcome of the proceedings. If the claim is indefensible, an apology has no real consequence save to possibly prevent a claim being brought. If the claim appears to be defensible or (as is often the case) it is impossible to tell, an apology can still be given, but care should be exercised in choosing the words. Try to ensure that the apology is a comment on what the complainant is saying rather than making a positive (adverse) comment about the hospital. Thus, saying you are sorry that the patient is distressed is preferable from a lawyer's viewpoint to saying that you are sorry for the distress that you have caused. The latter comment could be considered to be a statement about the causation of the complainant's condition, albeit an indirect one. Negligence without causation does not result in a successful claim. Keep to the facts and avoid opinions. Nevertheless, there can be no hard and fast rules and any sense of artificiality is likely to detract from the purpose of making the apology. Some helpful guidance on the issue of apologies, explanations and associated small offers of compensation, has recently been given by the NHS Litigation Authority. The circular talks in terms of sympathising with the patient or relatives and expressing sorrow or regret at the adverse outcome. Explanations of what has led to adverse outcomes is encouraged. It is emphasised that explanations should be based on facts and not opinions[75].

Similar concerns are voiced about the implications of keeping untoward clinical incident reports. These are often not actual errors but near misses (as discussed in Chapters 3 and 4). Will the documents be disclosable in subsequent court proceedings? What are the implications? The cost/benefit ratio needs to be considered.

For a full exposition of the rules on discovery of documents, reference should be made to Rules of the Court[76]. In essence, privilege can only be claimed if the dominant purpose of bringing the document into existence was litigation, either actual or contemplated. These documents by their nature will not be the subject of legal privilege. They are brought into being far too early on. To be disclosable a document has to be relevant to the proceedings. Therefore in an anaesthetic accident report forms relating to other incidents with the same anaesthetic may be disclosable, but report forms relating to all anaesthetic accidents should not. Is this a factor to take into consideration when deciding whether an untoward clinical incident reporting system is worthwhile? If the disclosure of these records leads the hospital to a previously unknown source of risk, the cost of having to settle the claim in hand could be quite small compared with the potential for repeat claims had the problem continued to go undiscovered.

If the patient has died there may be an inquest to attend. It should be borne in mind that this is a fact finding exercise rather than a means of establishing fault. The verdict of the coroner is not binding on either a civil or criminal court.

Care should be taken in preparing for the inquest. The coroner has the power to refer the file to the Director of Public Prosecutions for consideration of a charge of manslaughter by gross negligence. The witnesses should be aware of the rule against self-incrimination. If anything said in a document or orally in the coroner's proceedings would tend to incriminate the witness in a criminal trial the witness can be silent on the point. Copies of the witness statements for the coroner and the transcript of the inquest will be disclosable documents in any future civil proceedings. The statements can be put to the witness in cross-examination at a civil trial if evidence then is inconsistent with the statements. Statements should therefore be prepared with the same care as if the proceedings were a civil trial for damages and legal advice sought as appropriate. In a difficult case consideration should be given to instructing counsel and having a pre-inquest conference. The coroner will usually produce a list of witnesses. It is advisable to keep strictly to that list and only volunteer extra information if legal advice recommends it. The hospital press office should be kept fully informed so that the matter can be handled positively and sensitively at all times.

Information about incidents and claims is unlikely to be of much benefit if kept in isolation. To keep in control of matters, trends need to be tracked and the best way of doing this is by a suitable software package whereby the data about claims and incidents can be dovetailed. The same system should be capable of dealing with quality issues and the provision of financial information about the costs of both claims and legal representation.

REFERENCES

1. Powers, M. J. and Harris, N. H. (1994) *Medical Negligence*, 2nd edn. Butterworths: London.
2. Pippin v Sheppard 1822 11 Price 400.
3. AB and Others v Tameside and Glossop Health Authority 1997 8 Med LR 91.
4. Bolam v Friern Hospital Management Committee 1957 2 All ER 118.
5. Maynard v West Midlands Regional Health Authority 1985 1 All ER 635.
6. Bolitho v City and Hackney Health Authority 1997 4 All ER 771.
7. Anon (1997) The end of the Bolam Test? *Medical Law Monitor*, December.
8. Pollard v Crockard and The Board of Governors of the National Hospital for Nervous Diseases (Maida Vale) 22 January 1997 (unreported).
9. Wilsher v Essex Area Health Authority 1987 2 WLR 437.
10. McCandless v General Medical Council. *The Times*, 12 December 1995.
11. For further reading on causation see *Healthcare Risk Report*, **4**, (3), 12.
12. Barnett v Chelsea and Kensington Hospital Management Committee 1968 1 All ER 1068.

13. Reibl v Hughes, Supreme Court of Canada 1980 114 DLR (3d) 1.
14. R v Dixon. December 1995 Nottingham Crown Court (unreported).
15. Sidaway v The Royal Bethlem and Maudsley Hospital 1985 1 All ER 643.
16. Smith v Tunbridge Wells Health Authority 1994 5 Med LR 334.
17. Rogers v Whittaker 1993 4 Med LR 79.
18. re C (adult: refusal of medical treatment) 1994 1 WLR 290.
19. re T (adult: refusal of consent) 1993 Fam Law 27.
20. re B (a minor, wardship: medical treatment) 1981 1 WLR 1421.
21. re T (a minor, wardship: medical treatment) 1997 1 All ER 906.
22. Fox, M. and McHale, J. (1997) In whose best interests? *Modern Law Review*, **60,** 700.
23. re C (a minor: withdrawal of lifesaving treatment) *The Independent*, 11 December 1997.
24. s.8 Family Law Reform Act 1969.
25. re W (a minor: medical treatment) 1992 4 All ER 627.
26. Gillick v West Norfolk Area Health Authority 1985 3 All ER 402.
27. re R 1993 15 BMLR 72.
28. Airedale NHS Trust v Bland 1993 4 Med LR 39.
29. Frenchay Health Care and NHS Trust v S 1994 1 WLR 601.
30. Practice Note (Official Solicitor: Vegetative State) 1996 2 FLR 375.
31. Working Group of Royal College of Physicians, Chairman Sir Douglas Black (1996) *Journal of the Royal College of Physicians*, **30,** 119–121.
32. Royal College of Paediatrics and Child Health (1996 plus 1998 addendum) *Withholding or Withdrawing Life Saving Treatment in Children. A Framework for Practice*. RCPCH: London.
33. *Who Decides? Making Decisions on behalf of Mentally Incompetent Adults*. Cmnd 3808.
34. NLJ Practitioner. 1 November 1996 p.1580.
35. s 1(2) Mental Health Act 1983.
36. F v West Berkshire Health Authority 1990 2 AC 1.
37. Abbass v Kenney 1996 7 Med LR 47.
38. Bartley v Studd. *Daily Telegraph*, 12 July 1995, p.3.
39. In re D (medical treatment: consent) *The Times*, 14 January 1998.
40. (1993) *Decisions Relating to Cardiopulmonary Resuscitation*. Statement from the BMA and RCN in association with the Resuscitation Council (UK).
41. re R (S Buckinghamshire NHS Trust). May 1996 Fam Div (unreported).
42. re F (in utero) 1988 Fam 122.
43. re S (adult: refusal of medical treatment) 1992 4 All ER 671.
44. Royal College of Obstetricians and gynaecologists (1994) *Consideration of the Law and Ethics in relation to Court Authorised Obstetric Intervention*. RCOG: London.
45. Tameside and Glossop Acute Services Trust v CH 1996 1 FLR 762.
46. Norfolk and Norwich Healthcare Trust v W. 1996 2 FLR 613.
47. Rochdale Healthcare (NHS) Trust v C 1997 1 FCR 274.
48. St George's Healthcare -v- S AER 12 August 1988 673.
49. re L 1997 1 FLR 6.
50. re MB 1997 8 Med LR 217.
51. EL 97 (32).
52. Selfe v Ilford and District Hospital Management Committee 1970 114 SJ 935.
53. Newell v Goldberg 1995 6 Med LR 371.
54. Lybert v Warrington Health Authority 1996 7 Med LR 71.
55. HSG (92) 32.
56. Clinical Negligence Scheme for Trusts (1997) *Risk Management Standards and Procedures: Manual of Guidance*. CNST: Bristol.
57. HC (91) 2.
58. Early v Newham Health Authority 5 Med LR 214.
59. Lord Woolf MR *Access to Justice*. HMSO July 1996.

60. *Review of Civil Justice and Legal Aid.* Report to the Lord Chancellor by Sir Peter Middleton GCB, September 1997. LCD.
61. *Clinical Disputes Resolution Protocol.* Version 1 July 1998.
62. *Access to Justice. Clinical Negligence Cases: Proposed New Procedures.* A Consultation Paper. LCD.
63. HC (89) 20.
64. HSG (94) 11.
65. Headford v Bristol and District Health Authority 1995 PIQR 180.
66. s.2(1) Civil Evidence Act 1968.
67. s.3 Access to Health Records Act 1990.
68. Tarasoff v Regents of the University of California 1976 551 P (2d) 334.
69. s.2(1) Civil Evidence Act 1995.
70. Order 38 rule 2A, Rules of the Supreme Court 1981.
71. Department of Health, 12th March 1996 (68). Complaints. HMSO: London.
72. The Social Security (Recovery of Benefits) Act 1997.
73. The New Compensation Recovery Scheme: Goodwill Payments and Property Damage Claims.
74. Lord Chancellor (1998) *Access to Justice with Conditional Fees: A Consultation Paper.* Lord Chancellor's Department: London.
75. 97/C10: 6 November 1997.
76. Order 24 Rules of the Supreme Court 1981.

10 CLINICAL RISK MODIFICATION AND ETHICS

Lucy Frith

INTRODUCTION

In this chapter there will be an examination of the ethical implications of clinical risk management. One of the main aims of risk management is to reduce the risk of harm to patients. Such an aim can be seen as an expression of two well accepted ethical principles: promoting beneficence (doing good) and ensuring non-maleficence (doing no harm). At least initially, risk management can be seen to be an ethical enterprise. However, the practical implementation of clinical risk modification can raise complex ethical dilemmas. The most fundamental of these dilemmas will be seen to be the difficulty of ensuring both the welfare of the individual on the one hand, and the welfare of the wider community of patients on the other. This chapter examines how an understanding of the ethical issues raised by clinical risk modification could help in attaining a balance between these possibly competing claims.

RISK MANAGEMENT

Risk management could be seen as a response to the increase in medical litigation over the last 20 years. Initially, risk management was designed to reduce the cost of litigation but now the aims have been extended to reducing incidents of harm and improving the quality of care. Risk management programmes aim to improve the quality of care for all patients (as discussed in previous chapters.) However, as with any large institution or system, in trying to promote the interests of the majority, the interests of particular individuals within that system could be adversely affected. The main question is to what extent, in promoting the welfare of the majority – the greater good – risk management schemes could adversely affect the interests of the individual patient.

In exploring this question the first argument will be whether risk should be seen as a relative term: relative, that is, to the expected benefits of a procedure. As perceived benefits may differ from patient to patient it may not be possible to make generalised risk assessments that are equally valid for all patients. This analysis will be applied to treatment decisions and clinical guidelines, arguing that guidelines are based on such generalised risk assessments. Therefore it will be suggested that although this generalised risk assessment may be beneficial for the wider community as a whole, it may be prejudicial to the interests of particular patients.

We will then examine a possible solution to this problem: that of obtaining informed consent for procedures. Also discussed is that to protect the interests of the individual patient fully informed consent is not only ethically desirable but also invaluable for the practical success of clinical risk modification. Finally, consideration will be given to how clinical risk modification could affect the ability of a healthcare professional to safeguard the interests of the individual patient.

DEFINITION OF RISK

Risk can be usefully defined as the probability of a negative outcome. This negative outcome can be seen both in terms of the probability of it happening and the severity of the consequences if it does. What we are concerned with, for risk management, is unacceptable risk: a risk where the negative outcome outweighs the positive effect of an activity. For instance, about three million people in Britain undergo a general anaesthetic every year. Of these three million about 250–300 will die as a result of the anaesthetic. This is generally thought to be an acceptable risk. Here, although the negative consequence is severe – death – the likelihood is deemed so remote that it is seen as an acceptable risk to take. General anaesthetics are performed even for minor surgery. In this case relatively small benefits, such as a painless tooth extraction, are worth the risk because the probability of a negative outcome is very low. However, if the probability of a negative outcome is higher we may only wish to take such a risk if the expected benefit is itself higher. For example, an experimental new surgical technique with an unproven success rate might only be worth considering if it was the sole life-saving treatment available. In this instance the possible benefit would be high. However, we would not consider such a high-risk operation if it only promised a lower benefit such as removing an unsightly mole.

INESCAPABLE RISK

All medical treatments carry some inescapable risk. Hence, to calculate what is an acceptable risk the possible adverse affects have to be balanced against the expected benefits. If, therefore, agreement could be reached on the desired benefits of a procedure then agreement over acceptable levels of risk would be straightforward. However, different parties and individuals will have distinct conceptions of what they consider to be desirable benefits. For instance, in considering cosmetic surgery: the risk of the operation going wrong would not be offset by the expected benefit of a better appearance. However, many people would disagree and see such a risk as perfectly acceptable because they put a greater premium on the expected benefit. There may be many good reasons for wanting cosmetic surgery, but the point here is simply that people place different values on different outcomes.

This understanding of risk as a relative term has important practical and ethical implications. It is possible that what is meant by an acceptable or unacceptable risk could be seen differently by the hospital, the doctor or the patient. This possible difference in viewpoints could create ethical problems. There could be a fundamental division between the individual patient's concept of benefit and the hospital's concern for the welfare of all patients. The case of child B is an example this[1].

CASE STUDY: CHILD B

Child B, who was suffering from leukaemia, was refused a second transplant operation by Cambridge Health Authority. Her father challenged the decision in the High Court, it then went to the Appeal Court where the Health Authority's decision was upheld[1].

The interesting aspects of this case, for our purposes, are the different views of expected benefit and consequent risk that the three parties held. For the health authority, the primary issue was the relationship between the cost of the treatment and the expected benefit. The authority told the Appeal Court that it had refused treatment on the grounds that, in their view, it would not be an effective use of resources. The treatment cost of £75 000 was not justified by the predicted success rate which was very low: the expected benefit did not justify the large outlay of resources.

The doctor responsible for the patient explained the refusal of treatment in different terms. The doctor thought that the slim chance of success of the operation and the increased suffering it would cause during the last few weeks of her life were not in the patient's best interests. Here, for the doctor, the risk of harm to the patient outweighed the expected benefit.

For the child's father any chance, no matter how slim, of increasing his child's life expectancy was justified. Her father believed it was in her best interests to take that chance. Although the harm of the operation was great, the potential benefit of increasing life expectancy made that harm justifiable.

DIFFERING CONCEPTS OF RISK

In this case all three parties had a different conception of the risk of the transplant because they had a different approach to the assessment of the possible benefits. This demonstrates that the risk of the operation could not be put in objective terms. It depends on the viewpoints of the parties involved and what they consider to be the important benefits. Broadly, the three viewpoints could be divided into two categories: the Health Authority's utilitarian calculation of trying to promote the greatest good for the greatest number and the doctor's and father's concern for the welfare of the individual patient. Hence, there could be a fundamental split between a hospital's view of acceptable risk and that of the patient. While hospitals are concerned with promoting the overall benefit for the community as a whole, patients are simply concerned with what is in their own interests. In the case of Child B, what was best for her as an individual might not have been best for the hospital as a whole as it would have taken resources away from other patients. This clearly illustrates the possible tension that could exist between the greater good and the good of the individual patient.

CLINICAL GUIDELINES AND RISK

Having examined the possible differences in perceived benefit between the hospital and the patient, the chapter will then look specifically at one mechanism by which hospitals try to reduce general risk and promote the greater good: the formulation of clinical guidelines. There will be discussions about the fact that such guidelines, based on a conception of risk that is primarily concerned with promoting the greater good, could adversely affect the interests of the individual patient. The chapter will first give a brief outline of the rationale behind the introduction of clinical guidelines and then consider how these guidelines can affect patient care.

Part of the process of clinical risk modification is to assess systematically current practice and identify risky treatments[2].

> It is in the interests of trusts to introduce protocols and guidelines of good clinical practice to minimise harm to patients, enhance the quality of care, and enhance the quality of reaction should any harm befall the patient.

Hence, two of the central features of risk management are the review of existing protocols and guidelines, and the writing of guidelines in areas where they are lacking. Since April 1994 all trusts have to show that they have started to develop clinical guidelines[3]. The NHS executive stated that[4]:

> . . . on the advice of the Clinical Outcomes Group, [they have] begun to commend a selected number of high-quality guidelines.

By assessing current practice and eliminating harmful, risky or ineffective treatments from a Trust's portfolio, risk management is one mechanism of instigating an improvement in clinical care[5]. The rationale behind these guidelines is that of treating like cases as in the same way. This is because unwarranted variation in treating similar cases is seen as a core problem for healthcare[6].

However, treatments which produce the desired effect can differ from person to person. Even patients with identical manifestations of a particular disease could give different weight to various outcomes depending on personal taste, social and family situations, life priorities and so on. Brazier cites an example that illustrates this[7]:

> A woman is told that radical mastectomy will maximise her prospects of recovery from breast cancer. She knows that if she loses a breast her husband will leave her and she knows that psychologically she is unable to cope with the necessary mutilation.

Hence she opts for the marginally less 'safe' option of lumpectomy. She is concerned both with the success rate and the consequences for her life and relationships. Here the woman's risk/benefit calculation could be different from another patient's assessment. Another woman may choose a mastectomy as she is less concerned about losing a breast and wants the treatment that has a higher success rate. This illustrates that the treatment decision has to incorporate an assessment of both the clinical effectiveness of a treatment and how appropriate it is for that person. Therefore, the introduction of guidelines might preclude an individual assessment of what is best for that particular patient. When used in this way as a clinical risk modification tool to promote the greater good, guidelines incorporate an assessment of risk that is held to be the same for all patients. This could come into conflict with an individual's conception of desirable benefit and their own personal risk assessment.

However, supporters of clinical guidelines might argue against this view of the treatment process. They might argue that there are enough similarities between patients suffering from the same condition to see them as being members of the same patient group (in statistical language forming part of the same reference class of patient). Therefore, all that needs to be established is which group the patient belongs to and then the appropriate clinical guideline can be followed. Patrick Suppes, for example, has argued that a decision regarding the individual patient can be extrapolated from other cases. Even though patients may vary in many respects (age, wealth etc.)[8]:

> . . . the direct medical consequences and the direct financial cost of a given method of treatment are the most important consequences, and these can be evaluated by summing across the patients and ignoring more individual features.

Suppes is right in one respect. It may be possible to construct broad generalisations about patients' preferences for certain medical consequences. However, these would have to remain at a very broad level as many of the individual factors affecting these consequences are ignored. For example, financial cost may not be an issue for someone very wealthy, whereas for others even the cost of a simple prescription could be prohibitive. Others may value their life in so far as they are able to look after their children. Although it might be possible to ascertain the types of consequences that are, on the whole, most important, it is impossible to predetermine their respective value objectively.

Many authors have drawn attention to the importance of recognising that good outcomes must be seen as relative to the patient. Hopkins and Solomon illustrate this point with the example of the management of stroke patients. They say that the course of the treatment and the outcomes of rehabilitation cannot be predetermined because each person's disability is unique. Hence the therapist has to concentrate on the goals and needs of the particular patients[9].

PATIENT HOMOGENEITY

Guidelines rely on patient homogeneity, that is patients being very similar. In stroke rehabilitation, where patient variation is high, it is difficult to write a precisely defined clinical guideline. There are on the other hand areas of health-care where patient variation is much lower, the removal of wisdom teeth for example. When this is the case guidelines can be useful[10].

> In conditions such as day case surgery, a single patient record is easy to introduce. In an intensive care setting, where variations are more common, a pathway together with freehand documentation may be more suitable.

There may be areas where guidelines are more applicable, however, this should not be extended to areas of healthcare provision where guidelines may be inappropriate. Even when patients are suffering from the same condition guidelines should not be applied unthinkingly. Room should be made for the needs and wants of the patient to be accommodated. It could be argued that due to the individual nature of many treatment decisions, it could be difficult to produce guidelines that reflect each patient's treatment preferences.

CONSENT AND CLINICAL RISK MANAGEMENT

Given that clinical risk modification schemes, in both seeking to further the greater good and relying on universal assessments of risk, can adversely affect the welfare of the individual patient, we need to ask how the patient's interests can be protected within such schemes. (Consent has been discussed in further detail in Chapters 6, 8 and 9.)

One possible way of protecting the welfare of the individual is to ensure that the patient always gives informed consent to any procedure. Informed consent can play two roles in clinical risk modification schemes. First, it can perform an ethical role: it is ethically desirable to get informed consent both as a way of respecting the autonomy and safeguarding the best interests of the individual. To allow patients to make their own decisions about their healthcare – to respect autonomy – is one of the fundamental ethical requirements of medical practice. Consent is also one of the best ways of ensuring that the medical care given is in the best interests of the patient. It is thought that the individual concerned will be the best person to promote his/her own interests. Second, it can perform a pragmatic role in ensuring the success of clinical risk modification schemes in practice and it is, of course, a legal requirement that patients consent to any treatment or procedures they undergo. If patients make more fully informed decisions about their healthcare they will feel more positively about their care and will be less likely to make complaints.

Before considering how consent can be used to protect the individual's welfare there will be a focus on two of the main obstacles to consent performing this role; first, the limited healthcare options that are available to an individual and second, the difficulties in communicating information to patients. These will be considered in turn.

Limited treatment options

With the implementation of guidelines the patient is only offered a limited range of options. If the treatment that would most benefit the individual is not part of a hospital's treatment protocol then consent simply becomes the act of being able to accept or refuse one of a limited number of options. Consent in this context becomes a negative action, in that the act of consent can only be to refuse an option that might be inappropriate. It is not to positively choose an option which may be most beneficial to the patient. Such a refusal clearly does little to safeguard a patient's interests because it does not provide the desired treatment. For instance, a woman might want to have a home birth but finds that in her area there is not the community midwifery support to enable her to do this. She opts for a hospital birth, but one that allows her to go home a few hours after the delivery. It can be said that she consents to this hospital birth, but she has only been offered a limited range of options and has not received the kind of care she wanted.

Regarding these points, it could be countered that patients inevitably face a restricted range of the options in any large healthcare system. The general practitioner cannot refer the patient for a treatment if it is not offered by a local hospital trust. Therefore, when deciding what treatment is appropriate both patient and doctor are constrained by the options available. However, the worry with the introduction of guidelines is that the limited flexibility that currently exists may be reduced even further. This is because the rationale behind guidelines is to recommend the best treatment, based on the belief that it is possible to locate one best treatment, rather than seeing it as a relative concept: relative to the individual patient.

Information giving

The second difficulty with obtaining fully informed consent from patients will now be examined. If consent is to perform the function of safeguarding the welfare of the individual, then it must be fully, or at least adequately, based on a full understanding of relevant information about the treatment.

This raises the ethical dilemma of how much information to give a patient about the treatment (see Bludell's chapter for the legal perspective on this issue). On the one hand, it is argued that telling the patient about all aspects of the treatment, such as risks, side effects etc., might distress the patient unduly. If a patient becomes worried before undergoing a procedure it could prejudice the success of the treatment. Hence, it is argued that on the grounds of promoting beneficence for the patient, from an ethical point of view it is better not to tell the patient everything. On the other hand, it is argued that the patient should be fully informed about the treatment, because if patients do not receive all the information they will be unable to make an autonomous choice. Hence, on the grounds of promoting the autonomy of the patient all the information should be fully disclosed. Therefore, the doctor is faced with the problem of trying to act ethically, either by acting beneficently towards the patient or by trying to promote the patient's autonomy: each course of action justified by one principle appears to contravene the other.

This ethical dilemma is compounded by the practical problem with giving information: it is often very hard to explain the risks of a treatment to patients. This is for two reasons: first, patients may find it hard to understand complex medical information that it has taken the doctor years to accumulate. Second, the risks of a treatment for a particular patient are always uncertain and uncertainties are hard to communicate. For instance, in one trial, men with mild hypertension were randomly allocated either a thiazide (bendroflumethiazide), a betablocker (propranolol) or a placebo. Men given the thiazide were 20 times more likely than men on the placebo to be withdrawn from the trial due to impotence. After two years on the trial impotence was reported as a symptom of 23 per cent of the men taking thiazide[11]. Hence, when recommending a treatment for mild hypertension the doctor would have information from the trial on the possible side effects of thiazide. The doctor would not be able to state with certainty whether the patient would suffer from the side effect of impotence and would only be able to state the relative likelihood of that occurrence. Communicating this kind of information to patients is very difficult.

Bearing in mind these ethical and practical difficulties over information giving, how much information should be disclosed to the patient and what risks should be outlined? The case of Chatterton -v- Gerson [1981] All ER 257 illustrates the legal approach to this question. Miss Chatterton took a case against her doctor, arguing that she had not given informed consent to a surgical procedure because she had not been given information of all the possible risks involved in the treatment. Her action failed as the judge said that a consent to surgery was valid providing that the patient was[7]:

. . . informed in broad terms of the nature of the procedure which is intended.

Miss Chatterton then took a negligence action and this too failed. The judge found that although the doctor should have told her about the most common risks inherent in the procedure, he did not have to tell her every single risk there might be. The decision of how much to tell her should be made by taking into account[7]:

> the personality of the patient, the likelihood of misfortune and what in the way of warning is for the particular patient's welfare.

The case of Sidaway -v- Bethlem Royal Hospital Governors [1985] AC 871 further reiterates that the duty of disclosure is not fixed (see Chapter 9 for an elaboration of this case). These cases illustrate that there is no legal definition of precisely how much information should be given to the patient. In English law, generally, the reasonable professional standard of information giving is adopted. Thus, it is left to the professional to decide how much information should be given to the patient.

However, the courts will not always accept the reasonable professional standard of information giving, and one of the judges in the Sidaway case stated that, in certain cases:

> disclosure of a particular risk was so obviously necessary to an informed choice on the part of the patient that no reasonably prudent medical man would fail to make it.

This is further discussed in Chapter 9. This judgement encapsulates the idea that doctors should act reasonably as well as acting in accordance with a responsible body of medical opinion.

It is difficult, if not impossible, to set a definitive standard of how much information a particular patient should be given. However, it is argued that a move away from the reasonable professional standard of information giving towards a prudent patient standard, that is what the prudent patient would want to know, would be a better rule of thumb to adopt. The prudent patient standard would mean that the patient would be better informed as the prudent patient generally requires more information than the prudent professional sees fit to divulge. Enabling patients to make more fully informed decisions about their healthcare would respect their autonomy.

CONSENT AS A PROCESS

A practical way of implementing the ethical aim of increasing the level of information giving is in seeing consent as an ongoing process, rather than as simply an authorisation to accept the treatment at the beginning of the procedure.

One way of increasing the information given to patients is to use clinical guidelines. For instance, writing guidelines in consultation with patient groups will enable the guideline to incorporate patient views on treatments. Guidelines can then be distributed to patients. When patients enter hospital they can be given a copy of the clinical guidelines and this can indicate what should be happening during the course of their treatment. It will give them an informed basis on which to question and challenge their treatment provision. This model has been adopted by a Liverpool hospital. The guideline is explained to the patient and they usually have access to it during their stay in hospital[10]. The patients therefore have a document that they can refer back to at any stage and so do not have to take in all the information at the beginning of their treatment. Used in this way guidelines can be a useful aid to communication between patient and healthcarer. This will ensure that the consent the patient gives is based on a full understanding of what the treatment involves.

Further, the guideline can be used to monitor the treatment. If a variation takes place, this can alert the staff to possible problems and early action can be taken. If patients are aware of the expected progression of the treatment, then they have some idea of what they should be receiving and can tell the staff if anything is not going as planned. This could prevent serious problems developing and improve documentation and record keeping. By giving the patient a greater understanding and hence control over the treatment, minor complaints and dissatisfaction could be reduced. clinical risk modification schemes are designed to eliminate complaints even if they turn out to be groundless. Hence, increasing the amount of information given to the patient could keep the patient better informed and help to prevent complaints. The importance of information giving is exemplified by the following case.

CASE STUDY: THE SWOLLEN ARM

A complaint was made by a woman who had been admitted to hospital with blood clots on the lung and had been put on a drip of heparin. Later in the course of treatment her arm swelled up and woman was not told why the swelling had occurred. Although it was treated successfully, the woman complained because she thought the swelling had occurred as a result of the nurse not cleaning her wound properly.

Adhering to a strict legal standard of information giving, that of the prudent professional, would not have prevented this complaint as the doctor would have been able to argue that when the patient was admitted it was not prudent to inform her of the possible risks of the drip as this could have caused her further anxiety. The issue here is not whether the woman would have refused consent if she had been given this information as it is unlikely that she would have refused the treatment because it was life-saving. The issue is one of imparting information when the patient needs it and is ready to take it in. If consent had been seen as an ongoing process with information being given gradually and throughout the treatment, then she would have been told what was happening when the swelling occurred – that it was a normal side effect of a drip. Another way of providing the information would be to give the patient a written guideline on how her treatment should progress, indicating possible common side effects. However the information was given it would have both curbed her distress and avoided the likelihood of her making a complaint.

Although consent can only go part of the way to protect the welfare of the individual patient, due to limited treatment options and the difficulties in information giving, it is still an essential part of ethical medical practice. It is important to ensure that the individual chooses between options freely and makes this decision on the basis of all the relevant information.

PROFESSIONAL ETHICAL ISSUES

Having concentrated on the implications of risk management for the individual patient, consideration will be given to the role the healthcare professional can play in risk management schemes. It is the responsibility of the healthcare professional to promote the welfare of individual patients and ensure that they receive the best care. First, consideration as to how risk management schemes affect this ethical duty will be discussed. Examination will be undertaken to see how such schemes can be used to create an environment which makes it easier for professionals to carry out their ethical duties in practice, looking at the issues of near-miss reporting and professional competence.

PROFESSIONAL AUTONOMY

The professional codes of conduct for doctors and nurses all state the ethical duties of the professional in terms of the duties to the individual patient. *The UKCC Professional Code of Conduct* (1992) states[12]:

> . . . act, at all times, in such a manner as to safeguard the interests of individual patients.

Doctors are bound by similar dictates to consider the welfare of the individual patient as paramount. Professional autonomy could be jeopardised if professionals felt that adhering to the guideline was inappropriate in a particular situation and were unable to deviate from it. Hence it is possible, at least in theory, that a professional's action could be acceptable to the hospital but contravene professional codes in respect of the ethical duty to do what is best for the individual patient.

The importance of this issue will depend on how binding the guidelines are within the hospital. If the hospital obliges the practitioners to sign a contract that requires compliance with the hospitals' clinical guidelines, then this might prevent them from exercising their clinical judgement regarding what is best for the individual patient. However, as Tingle states[13,14]:

Patient and healthcarer choice are factors which clearly impact on the *appropriateness* (as discussed by Wilson: 1996)[13] of the application of the clinical guideline. Some clinical guidelines in the USA have written warnings on the front of them stating that they must not be automatically applied and that the clinical judgement of the healthcarer must always be exercised first.

An example of the needs of one patient not being met by the strict application of a clinical guideline, is the case of Wickline -v- State of California 1986, cited by Tingle[14]. The California Medicaid programme (Medi-Cal) refused a doctor's request for additional days of patient monitoring on the grounds that they were not required under the clinical algorithms developed by Medi-Cal. The patient was discharged and developed complications. She sued Medi-Cal for negligence, arguing that she had been discharged solely on the grounds of cost. The court ruled in her favour saying physicians should not disregard good medical judgement for cost reasons. Thus it has been argued that[14]:

> . . . care paths must be scientifically based and never distorted solely to effect cost control or other non-scientific support.

The way that guidelines are used in the hospitals will determine how much variance is allowed and on what grounds. For instance, there could be space on the documentation for freehand comments to justify the variance from the guideline. It is also important to set out on what grounds variance would be allowed. For example, would a change in treatment from that recommended by the guideline be allowed on the grounds of patient preference? This is an important question in terms of how far the professional is able to go in safeguarding or promoting the welfare of a particular patient.

If clinicians are given a significant say in the writing and formulation of guidelines, this should further reduce possible infringements of professional autonomy and allow professionals to care for their patients as they think fit. This raises the issue of the overriding rationale for guidelines. If they are primarily designed to eliminate risky and costly treatments from a hospital's range of services then the guidelines produced could be very different from those written by clinicians who are concerned primarily with patient care. As mentioned earlier, to ensure that both the needs of the individual and the wider community are met, a balance needs to be struck. To this end guidelines should be formulated by a consensus of all the interested parties.

The adoption of clinical guidelines by a hospital does not in itself pose a threat to the exercise of professional autonomy. It is the way in which guidelines are used in practice that will determine how much restriction they place on medical staff.

NEAR-MISS REPORTING: AN ETHICAL ENVIRONMENT

One aspect of risk management that can be used as an important measure for preventing harm to patients is near-miss reporting (as discussed in Chapters 3, 4 and 9). This could be used to create a working environment which helps the professional to practise ethically. The hospital appoints a risk manager to compile information on accidents or possible accidents which forms the basis of changes designed to protect the patient from further incidents. This mechanism can improve patient care and is a means by which risk management can promote ethical practice. As Professor Jones says[2]:

> It cannot be ethical to continue with a method of providing healthcare that exposes patients to unacceptable risks of having an adverse outcome.

This move by the medical profession to examine why medical accidents have occurred is a very positive trend. For example, studies that focus specifically on such issues, such as the work of Ennis and Vincent who examined obstetric accidents, can help to highlight problematic areas of practice and reduce harm to patients[15].

Clearly any reduction in processes leading to patient harm, incidents of staff incompetence and general bad practice are to be applauded. However, there could be a potential difficulty with this approach when one considers the context in which it operates. Lyon has argued that, in order for an adequate system of near-miss reporting to operate, the staff must be able to trust their employer to use the information responsibly[16]. As recent cases demonstrate this might not always be so. For example, a nurse was employed to manage a purpose-built unit for elderly mentally ill patients, which had not yet been built. He complained to the trust that there were faults in the design and consequently the building would be unsafe for staff and patients. The trust ignored his complaints and later made him redundant. Although an industrial tribunal upheld his claim for unfair dismissal he had still lost his job. As a result of reporting a possible risk the nurse had effectively been dismissed. The NHS reforms have, according to some, created a culture of fear[17]:

> A survey published by the union, Manufacturing Science Finance, and published in February 1993, showed that fear of losing their jobs was keeping NHS staff from talking to the media about malpractice and poor standards.

Staff members could feel threatened by having to report mistakes and accidents to the risk manager. The NHS Executive has stated that[4]:

> . . . the results of the risk management process should not be used for punitive or disciplinary purposes.

It also states that the information given should be kept confidential and that the informant should remain anonymous. Such confidentiality could ensure that the near-miss reporting scheme could effectively carry out the stated aims. This would be beneficial to both staff and patients and ensure that the ethical aims of risk management schemes could be realised. As long as the possible fears of the staff are borne in mind by employers, a culture of trust could be fostered and non-punitive mechanisms developed for addressing the concerns of employees.

THE BAD DOCTOR

A specific problem clearly arises when a healthcarer is reporting a colleague who is allegedly incompetent. It could be argued that near-miss reporting schemes that ensure that the information source would be kept confidential would encourage people to report possible incidents of incompetence. The General Medical Council stipulates that it is a doctor's duty to inform the appropriate authority about a colleague whose performance is questionable. The UKCC also has requirements in its code of conduct that nurses should:

> . . . report to an appropriate person or authority any circumstances in which safe and appropriate care for patients cannot be provided.

The appropriate response to an allegation of incompetence clearly depends on the type of accident or incompetence that is reported. Serious misconduct or wilfully disregarding the welfare of the patient should merit disciplinary action. The issue that is of more concern here is a genuine accident or mistake that the practitioner did not wilfully cause. Whether the accident was caused by a lack of skill or an inadequate process, these factors should be able to be addressed without the practitioner facing any form of disciplinary procedure. In this way risk management schemes can be used to create a more ethical environment in which to practise. If near-miss reporting is not used for punitive purposes but generally to help improve patient care then the reporting of incompetent colleagues could be done against the background of helping them rather than with an eye to disciplinary action.

CONCLUSION

The central theme of this chapter has been the difficulty in trying to ensure both the welfare of the individual and the welfare of the wider community of patients. This chapter has demonstrated that ethical principles can be used by risk management schemes to formulate practical ways of representing the interests of the individual patient and promoting the interests of the greater good by reducing litigation.

The central problem is that the promotion of the interests of the individual patient has implications for the interests of the greater good. If an individual consumes large amounts of medical resources this could be said to be a form of indirect harm to the wider community. It is a well-accepted principle, in law at least, that individual freedom of action can be restricted on the grounds that it harms others[18]. Hence, by promoting the interests of one individual, others may suffer. However, the other extreme where individual priorities have no place in healthcare delivery should not be adopted. Clearly, there needs to be some balance struck between ensuring the welfare of the wider community of patients on the one hand and the welfare of particular individuals on the other.

Within a large healthcare system provision should be made for the individual to exercise as much choice as possible, recognising that this choice might be constrained by available resources and the needs of others. Risk management schemes if properly implemented could help facilitate this balance.

REFERENCES

1. R -v- Cambridge HA exp B (a minor) 1995 23 BMLR 1 CA.
2. Jones, M. (1997) *Clinical Risk Management*. pp. 8, 12. IMLAB Publication, Liverpool.
3. DoH (1992) *A Vision for the Future*. HMSO: London.
4. NHS Executive (1994) *Risk Management in the NHS*. p. 20. HMSO: London.
5. Kitchiner, D. *et al.* (1995) Integrated care pathways. *Journal of Evaluation in Clinical Practice*, **2**, 65–69.
6. James, B. (1993) Implementing practice guidelines through clinical quality improvement. *Frontiers of Health Service Management*, **10**, 3–37.
7. Brazier, M. (1992) *Medicine, Patients and the Law*. pp. 78, 82, 88. Penguin: Harmondsworth.
8. Suppes, P. (1979) The logic of clinical judgement: Bayesian and other approaches. p. 151 in *Clinical Judgment: A Critical Appraisal* (H.T. Engelhardt, S.F. Spicker and B. Towers, eds). Reidel Publishing Company.
9. Hopkins, A. and Solomon, J. K. (1996) Can contacts drive clinical care? *British Medical Journal*, **313**, 477–8.
10. Kitchiner, D. and Bundred, P. (1996) Integrated care pathways. *Archives of Disease in Childhood*, **75**, 166–168.
11. Sackett, D., Haynes, B., Guyatt, G. and Tugwell, P. (1991) *Clinical Epidemiology: A Basic Science For Clinical Medicine*. Little, Brown: Boston.
12. United Kingdom Central Council for Nurses, Midwives and Health Visitors (1992) *Professional Code of Conduct*. UKCC: London.
13. Wilson, J. H. (1996) *Integrated Care Management: The Path to Success*. Butterworth-Heinemann: Oxford.
14. Tingle, J. (1996) Clinical guidelines: risk management and legal issues. *British Journal of Nursing*, **5**, (5), 266–7.
15. Ennis, M. and Vincent, C. (1990) Obstetric accidents. *British Medical Journal*, **300**, 1365.
16. Lyon, J. (1996) *The Trojan Horse: Problems of Clinical Risk Management*. MSc Dissertation, University of Liverpool.
17. Hunt, J. (ed.) (1995) *Whistleblowing in the Health Service*. Edward Arnold: London.
18. Feinberg, J. (1973) *Social Philosophy*. Prentice-Hall: London.

11 CONCLUSIONS AND THE WAY FORWARD

Jo Wilson and John Tingle

CONCLUSIONS

In this book the authors have sought to reveal and discuss the substance of clinical risk management and the importance of clinical risk modification. The emphasis is on evolution, not revolution, as culture and behaviour take time and effort to change. The discipline has been seen in both academic and practical contexts and is clearly reflective of both. The issues discussed have been wide ranging, from substantive medical law in Cheryl Blundell's and Paul Balen's chapters, practical application with the importance of data and information in Jo Wilson's and Denny Van Liew's chapters, to Lucy Frith's discussions of the ethics involved in clinical risk modification. What is clear from all of the discussions in the book is that clinical risk management is needed, is relevant to everyday NHS activities and has a future. Clinical risk modification practices are helping all healthcare providers, insurers and commissioners of care to focus on quality and the causes of complaints and litigation. Reflective clinical practices, achieved through such techniques as clinical guidelines, integrated care and Multidisciplinary Pathways of Care©, are helping to ensure that evidence-based practice, consistent standards, appropriate patient care and good clinical outcomes are attained.

There have been many references to the 1997 NHS reforms, and we make no apologies for this, as there is therein a strong emphasis on providing seamless care which is consistent with high-quality standards and good clinical outcomes. The government White Paper makes explicit the link between clinical risk modification and clinical governance[1]. It aims to ensure that care is provided by highly trained, competent staff who can meet and maintain performance levels in the best interest of the patient. The aim is to concentrate on health promotion as well as commissioning and targeting care to where patient needs are greatest. The use of integrated care and health improvement programmes will help to ensure that care and practices are appropriate to patient needs and expectations. The White Paper includes among the practices that a quality organisation will have to ensure, requirements that:

. . . clinical risk reduction programmes of a high standard are in place . . .

and

. . . lessons for clinical practice are systematically learned from complaints by patients.

Complaints have been well covered within this book from the patient's and carer's perspectives. It is necessary for patients to take more responsibility for healthcare by attending appointments, having a better understanding of how the services work to their benefit, and not abusing services. The new Patient's Charter which is currently being prepared will set out the standards of treatment and care that patients can expect from the NHS and explain in detail patient's rights and responsibilities. Healthcare professionals must begin to incorporate patient requirements, needs and realistic expectations by asking patients/clients what they want, learning from them about what works well, and prioritising quality improvement projects to promote high-quality, low-risk and cost-effective care. The professional's definition of quality may be quite different from the client's and what is high-quality healthcare today may not be one year from now. Thus the need for constant, ongoing evaluation from the patient and provider becomes critical to the overall success of the clinical risk modification programme.

CLINICAL GOVERNANCE AND CLINICAL RISK

Clinical risk modification is an important feature of clinical governance. With the implementation of the 1997 White Paper[1] new statutory duties (subject to legislation) have been imposed on all healthcare providers to participate in local health plans and health improvement programmes (HIPS) through consultation, partnership, cooperation, communication and integrated care management (ICM)[2]. NHS organisations also have, for the first time, a statutory responsibility (subject to legislation by parliamentary approval) to work in partnership and to maintain and improve the quality of care they provide, by processes which are subject to external scrutiny, review and accountability. From April 1999 all healthcare providers will have to guarantee quality of care through a new process called clinical governance. This incorporates clinical audit; evidence-based practice; clinical effectiveness; clinical risk management; monitoring outcomes of care; and clinical risk reduction programmes. Clinical governance places a duty of responsibility on the chief executive, trust board and all healthcare professionals to ensure that care is satisfactory, consistent and responsive. Individuals will be responsible for the quality of their clinical practice as part of professional self-regulation.

Clinical governance processes

The following steps must be taken to ensure the realisation of clinical risk modification and quality of care:

- clinical quality improvements integrated with clinical risk modification and continuous quality improvement programmes to identify and build upon good practice;
- good practice systematically disseminated;
- clinical risk reduction and risk review programmes;
- professional self-regulation/assessment, including the development of clinical leadership skills;
- evidence-based practice systems;
- adverse events, near misses and incidents detected, openly investigated and lessons learned;
- complaints to be dealt with positively and the information used to improve the organisation and care delivery;
- high quality and performance measurement data collected to monitor clinical care and support professionals in the delivery of that care;
- poor clinical performance dealt with appropriately to minimise harm to patients and other staff;
- staff should be supported in their duty to report concerns about colleagues' professional conduct and performance;
- continuing professional development and life-long learning aligned with clinical governance principles.

These processes will ensure proper mechanisms are in place for continually monitoring and improving clinical quality. There need to be clear lines of responsibility and accountability for the overall quality and clinical risk modification of clinical care. Every healthcare organisation will be required to produce their first clinical governance report for external review in spring 2000.

THE LAW

The law has also been closely linked with clinical governance. There will be a legal duty of quality imposed on every hospital in England for the first time in the history of the NHS[3]. The new statutory duty will be put into place, subject to legislation, in 1999. Quality is now the prime directive for the NHS and as such clinical risk management practices will be playing a fundamental role.

The law provides the framework for the resolution of disputes in healthcare where compensation is sought and as such directly influences the culture of clinical practice. The law cannot be ignored.

We have seen that complaints and legal claims stand at record levels. This promotes controversy and soul searching on how to improve matters. The Health Secretary, Frank Dobson, has made the following comments, which some lawyers consider to be quite justified. In a *Times* news item he was reported as saying to the Royal College of Midwives[4]:

> As far as I am concerned, the best place for lawyers in the NHS is on the operating table, not sliding around causing trouble for other people.

There are a number of causes of litigation and complaints in healthcare and it is clear, as Lord Woolf stated in his report, that[5]:

> [Legal] proceedings often start because the claimant cannot get the information he is seeking, or an explanation or apology, from the doctor or the hospital. Historically, solicitors have had no alternative but to advise legal action, which is unlikely to be appropriate in all cases unless the client's main or only objective is to obtain financial compensation.

Many lawyers will argue that the main problem in healthcare complaints and litigation is that of communication failure (as discussed in Chapter 2). So if we improve patient communication strategies there will be less complaints and litigation. Urgent improvements need to be made to the way healthcarers talk to patients[6] and to aspects of record keeping in the NHS[7]. Successful communication is at the heart of creating an image of kind and concerned healthcare professionals. Communication has an intimate bearing on how healthcare providers are perceived and whether healthcare organisations are thought of as caring. Clinicians who apply positive communication techniques to their interactions with patients create a caring relationship; those who also extend support to staff enhance others' self-esteem and create a better workplace environment. Therefore, proper attitudes and the ability to communicate are vital to the quality, economic and risk management success of a healthcare organisation.

Lord Woolf put the issue of NHS litigation neatly in perspective and focus when he gave his reasons for looking at clinical negligence[5], as highlighted in Chapter 1. He pointed to the fact that unmeritorious cases are often pursued, and clear cut claims defended for too long. He also pointed to the fact that suspicion between the parties is more intense and the lack of cooperation greater than in many other areas of litigation. A culture change is called for and that is what is needed to change practices and behaviour.

CULTURE CHANGE

A change in NHS litigation will come about with the Woolf reforms, the proposed changes to legal aid funding of clinical negligence cases[8] and the NHSLA panel of solicitor changes. We are also going to see the dawning of the new specialist lawyers. It is worrying when looking at clinical negligence cases closed by the legal aid board in 1996/97 that in only 17 per cent of cases was £50 or more recovered[5]. The report states:

> Medical negligence cases are a specialist area of litigation. It can be difficult to identify at the outset whether a case has merit, and even as the medical evidence unfolds whether the negligence alleged has caused the ailment or injury. The government believes that part of the reason for the high failure rate is that cases are being pursued by lawyers who are insufficiently

experienced in this area of litigation. They do not have the experience or knowledge to identify at or from the outset cases which have little merit, nor can they properly appraise the evidence of medical reports that would allow them to stop cases sooner.

The government proposes to limit the right of choice of solicitor who may undertake clinical negligence cases under legal aid. The NHSLA have also formed a panel of defendant solicitors who can act for trusts under the CNST[9].

THE NET RESULT

The net result of this central government driven specialist lawyer focus should be to drive up the quality of clinical negligence professional legal services and to save public money. Those lawyers who take cases on conditional fees are already having to practise a form of legal risk management and identify at the outset a case that is likely to succeed. If they take on weak cases they will soon tie up essential resources and meet severe difficulties in carrying out their legal practice. Risk management for lawyers is now in vogue.

THE COMMON LAW AND THE SPECIALIST LAWYER

The common law is also forcing health lawyers to become more medically literate and experts will have to do a risk analysis and their reports will have to be more carefully reasoned and referenced as Foster argues when discussing the House of Lords case of Bolitho -v- City and Hackney Health Authority (1998)[10].

Lord Brown-Wilkinson in Bolitho when talking about the Bolam principle and expert opinion stated:

> The use of these adjectives responsible, reasonable and respectable all show that the court has to be satisfied that the exponents of the body of opinion relied upon can demonstrate that such opinion has a logical basis. In particular in cases involving, as they so often do, the weighing of risks against benefits, the judge before accepting a body of opinion as being responsible, reasonable or respectable, will need to be satisfied that, in forming their views, the experts have directed their minds to the questions of comparative risks and benefits and have researched a defensible conclusion on the matter.

Risk analysis and evidence-based practice will feature more strongly in medical literature as Foster demonstrates in his analysis of Bolitho[10]. More medically literate lawyers and judges will become more probing in looking at expert medical and nursing practices and will be increasingly looking at the basis of clinical decision making. As Foster argues, the recent GMC Inquiry about Bristol Royal Infirmary shows how audit data can be used and wielded in a quasi-litigious forum. Audit data, clinical guidelines and evidence-based practice may become regular features in cases. The role and link between clinical risk modification and the law can be seen to be firmly established.

CLINICAL RISK MODIFICATION THROUGH BEST-PRACTICE GUIDELINES

Best-practice guidelines and MPCs[©2] are rapidly becoming an established and essential feature of modern day clinical practice. They help to facilitate a process of ensuring consistency, collaboration and communication of care delivery, to reduce clinical variations, and to provide the best defensibility (not defensive medicine) if things do go wrong by demonstrating a controlled environment of care delivery. They can be seen in a wide variety of clinical settings ranging right across the primary, secondary and tertiary health and social care spectrums. The 1997 White Paper[1] has a strong emphasis on quality and consistency of care delivery with assurances of performance measurements, integrated care[2] and clinical governance. It suggests making healthcare delivery against national standards a local responsibility, making quality of care the driving force for decision making at every level of the service, to ensure excellence for patients no matter where the care is provided. A number of controversial issues surround the use of guidelines. Some argue that guidelines are a fetter on clinical discretion and freedom and can lead to the practice of 'cookbook medicine'. Others maintain that best-practice guidelines are an essential aid to providing safe and appropriate medical and nursing care. There are arguments both for and against the use of best-practice guidelines.

Best-practice guidelines are[2]:

> . . . systematically developed statements which assist clinicians and patients in making decisions about appropriate treatment of specific conditions.

They originate through professional organisations, evidence-based practices and locally tailored interdisciplinary agreements based on local research. They are meant to be a guide to share best practice, but are no substitute for professional judgement or individual accountability. The knowledge, education, skills and competencies must be used to apply them appropriately, as they should not be applied slavishly or automatically; practitioners are still responsible and accountable for the practices they deliver. They are broad statements of principle giving practical guidance and consensus agreement assisting in decision making on the path to follow to achieve acceptable outcomes. Best-practice guidelines usually suggest a course of action with elements which are both optional and mandatory and they assist in the maintenance of patient and staff safety.

The Department of Health (DOH) is also actively encouraging the development and use of best-practice guidelines as Winyard states[11].

Clinical guidelines provide a key vehicle for promoting evidence-based practice and a basis for systematic audit. That is why they are so important. The NHS . . . with the active participation of the professions, has developed a strategy which aims for evidence-based clinical guidelines not just being used by clinicians, but also other partners in care – patients, purchasers, providers, indeed everyone who is involved to some degree in the decision making process.

Best-practice guidelines are fast becoming an increasing and established feature of the care environment. The NHS executive good practice booklet on clinical guidelines[17] establishes criteria by which guidelines should be appraised:

- valid – leading to results expected of them;
- reproducible – given the same evidence and methods of guideline development, another group of developers will come up with the same results;
- reliable – given the same clinical circumstances different health professionals interpret and apply the guidelines in the same way;
- cost effective – leading to improvements in health at acceptable costs;
- representative – by involving the contribution of key groups and interests in their development;
- clinical applicability – patient populations or services affected are unambiguously defined;
- flexible – by identifying exceptions to recommendations as well as the patient preferences to be used in decision making;
- clear – unambiguous language is used and readily understood by clinicians and patients;
- revisable – the date and process of review will be stated; and
- amenable to clinical audit – should be capable of translation into explicit audit criteria.

Properly constructed, appraised, best-practice guidelines have the potential to reduce complaints and litigation levels in healthcare by improving channels of communication, promoting integrated seamless care and having all professionals involved. When best-practice guidelines are utilised with staff having the necessary education, training, skills and competencies to apply them in a meaningful and professional way, the quality of care should be improved with a reduction in clinical risk exposure. This should lead to better risk modification with clearly defined practices, higher quality of care and less patient injuries or unexpected or unwanted outcomes. By adopting clinical risk management strategies such as best-practice guideline and clinical pathway developments, the quality of patient care can be improved. The process of identifying and documenting best practices helps to identify variations and weak areas of clinical practice.

CONCLUSIONS

The demand for providing high-quality, clinically and cost effective healthcare has never been greater. The clinical risk modification process is a dynamic one which will evolve further with better evaluation, sharing and benchmarking of best-practice guidelines, clinical indicators and regular patient record reviews against standards and outcomes of patient care. The future looks bright in terms of being able to use this data for assessing performance measurement and quality, enhanced patient and staff safety, and clinical and cost effectiveness for better resource utilisation. Data sources are going to be dynamic and ongoing sources of qualitative and quantitative information. Using this data appropriately will help to outline areas for quality improvements, potential risk exposures and areas of practice deficiencies. This will help to meet the Government's objective of an NHS which delivers fairer provision of services, higher quality, improved value for money, greater responsibility and thereby better health. The Government is committed to ensuring that the way in which performance of healthcare delivery is assessed and managed fully reflects the service's overall goals and objectives.

The next few years are going to be challenging times for all healthcare providers. The requirement to improve the quality of clinical care and to reduce clinical risk exposure means greater clinical responsibilities and accountabilities. Clinicians need to work in partnership with managers to improve patient care and ensure effective decision making. Good clinical care is care that is appropriate for the patient who needs it. By providing optimum care for the right people at the right time, in the right place, with the right people with the right skills and competency levels, not only will patients' health improve, but there will also be a reduction in the rate of complications and unwanted outcomes due to ineffective or substandard care. The way forward has to be fully utilising ways of ensuring consistency in practice, reduced clinical variability, evidence-based medicine, best-practice guidelines, clinical effectiveness and demonstrable quality of patient care with better ICM. These will all make a clinical risk modification system which is important for clinical, financial, business and organisational risk management.

Clinical governance will have an important part to play in restoring public confidence in healthcare delivery. Patients and their families place trust in healthcare professionals and they need to be assured that their treatment is up to date, and clinically and cost-effectively applied by staff whose skills have kept pace with evidence-based practice and new techniques. The emphasis must be on processes and systems that are simple to use and are able to demonstrate the production of effective results. It must be seen as going hand in glove with clinical risk management in terms of modifying the healthcare provider's behaviour in order to provide safe, effective and high quality care delivery. Quality and risk are two sides of the same coin and they must work in synergy together with the legal system to provide better patient care. Effective clinical governance and clinical risk modification will make it clear that quality is everyone's business.

REFERENCES

1. Department of Health (1997) *The New NHS, Modern, Dependable.* Cmnd 3807. HMSO: London.
2. Wilson, J. H. (1996) *Integrated Care Management: The Path to Success.* Butterworth-Heinemann: Oxford.
3. Department of Health (1998) Press Release 98/141, 13 April 1998 NHS to have a legal duty of ensuring quality for the first time. DOH: London.
4. *The Times*, 30 April 1998.
5. Lord Woolf (1996) *Access to Justice: Final Report.* HMSO: London.
6. Royal College of Physicians (1997) *Improving Communications between Doctors and Patients.* The Royal College of Physicians of London.
7. Department of Health (1998) *Improving Clinical Communications.* Clinical Systems Report. HMSO: London.
8. Lord Chancellor (1998) *Access to Justice with Conditional Fees: A Consultation Paper.* Lord Chancellor's Department: London.
9. National Health Service Litigation Authority. (1998) Letter 4/98. NHSLA.
10. Foster, C. (1998) Bolam: consolidation and clarification. *Healthcare Risk Report*, **4**, (5), 1998, 5–7.
11. Winyard, G. (1995) Improving clinical effectiveness: a coordinated approach. In *Clinical Effectiveness from Guidelines to Cost Effective Practice* (M. Hitch and S Hitch, eds). Earlybrave: Essex.
12. NHS Executive (1996) *Clinical Guidelines.* DOH: Leeds.

INDEX